Intermittent Fasting Book

The Proven Method for Achieving Longevity, Efficient Weight Loss, and Optimal Health

Olivia Rivers

Table of Contents

Introduction to Intermittent Fasting

"Intermittent fasting" is everywhere these days, isn't it? Our friends are trying it, and our families. We have probably heard of celebrities and celebrity doctors who are doing it, recommending it, or both.

But what is it? Does it work? And, if it does, how and to what extent?

Let's start from the top, then. Intermittent fasting is exactly what it sounds like: cycling between eating and fasting, throughout the day or even throughout the week. In other words, there are periods when you choose not to eat, with the goal that, in doing so, you lay claim to a whole host of health benefits.

And what are these benefits? Without spoiling the remainder of the book, let's just say that practicing intermittent fasting can help with weight loss, diabetes, and a whole list of other health issues. And it is as easy as consciously carving out a portion of your day where you just do not eat.

The problem is that we have all heard claims like this before. We know about the fad diets, the one-size-fits-all cures that are supposed to make us lean overnight. A list of these would be endless, but suffice it to say that on top of all the ones that have taken off, there are probably countless more that have not.

So, what makes intermittent fasting so different? Why is it not just another case of a supposedly simple way toward healthy living that winds up being either (a) totally made up; or (b) actually super bad for you?

Well, to answer that we will have to go back to the beginning of medicine itself, because it turns out that fasting has been recommended as a tool for healthy living since at least the time of Ancient Greece.

Hippocrates and the Origins of Fasting

The so-called Father of Medicine is a man named Hippocrates II. He lived on an island called Kos between 460 and 370 BCE—a long time ago. And yet, his contributions to medicine are so important that, even today, doctors take what is called the Hippocratic Oath—essentially, a promise by doctors to uphold certain ethical standards.

Of course, since he was the first medical doctor, there are lots of things about his practice that would seem odd to us today. For example, he said that yawning could be cured by a mixture of wine and water and that sneezing happens because our heads are too hot (Hippocrates, 2015). And when we look back on the history of medicine as a whole, we find strange practices like bloodletting, the theory that depression was caused by "black bile," and many more that today we would understand as barbaric and with zero basis in fact.

But one curious entry in the work of Hippocrates reads thus: "Fasting should be prescribed to those who have humid flesh; for fasting dries bodies" (Hippocrates, 2015).

Okay, so what does that mean? What is he referring to when he says people can have "humid flesh"? And does fasting actually dry bodies?

The truth is, I have no idea what it means to have humid flesh. I could think of a number of possibilities, but we are talking about a book that was written super long ago and that definitely references a whole bunch of conditions that seem alien to us today. And, as for fasting drying bodies, Lord knows where he got that from.

But let's take a step back here: No matter what condition he was referring to, Hippocrates understood that there was a place for fasting in the treatment of some ailments. Right at the beginning of medicine, fasting was a part of the conversation.

But while some theories went the way of the dodo, fasting has curiously stuck around. And not merely as a medical practice either: Many of our religious traditions still observe periods of fasting.

Fasting as a Spiritual Exercise

Consider the season of Lent in Christianity. Famous for being a period of fasting, in the Middle Ages this season was way more extreme than it is now. For example, on Good Friday, Christians were only allowed to eat one meal, which consisted of bread and water just after sunset. Nowadays, millions of Catholics in particular continue to observe Lent as a time of stripping oneself of excess and engaging in a 40-day fast.

But for what reason? Simply put, it is a time of spiritual purification, a kind of training, military-style, for the soul—like Travis Bickle in *Taxi Driver*. Fasting in this way is understood to make you sharper, stronger, and more attuned to your nature. You become "holier" through the process as you gain more self-control.

The practice is similar in all kinds of religions, from Islam to Buddhism. And all with at least a similar goal of improving your spiritual life.

Fasting and Health

Okay, fine, but this book is not a spiritual guide. It's a health book, right?

Yes. Of course. But let's think about this for a second: Setting aside our religious or spiritual inclinations, the notion that fasting is a part of a healthy lifestyle has lasted a long, long time. And whether our ancestors were right or wrong about the way in which the practice is healthy, they understood that it was at least healthy in some way. Fasting, in other words, did not go the way of bloodletting because there seems to be something to it. Something, maybe, that we are just beginning to learn about now.

And, believe me, we are definitely learning about it now. Because as we have discovered more about the body, we have also learned more about which kinds of fasting—the "methods" or "protocols"—work the best.

We will be getting into these in more detail later but for now, suffice it to say, there are a bunch of different fasting protocols you can use or experiment with. For example, there is the 16:8 method, where you skip breakfast and only eat between 1 p.m. and 9 p.m., thereby fasting for 16 hours. Then there is the Eat Stop Eat method, where you do not eat for 24 hours once a week (say, from dinner one day to dinner the next). And then there's the 5:2 diet, where you pick two consecutive days a week to only eat between 500 and 600 calories, then eat normally on the other days.

Of course, there are plenty more too. But even just sticking with these, we will find that some people are more attuned to one type of fasting or another, or they may want to experiment and try another one out after they have gotten used to a particular type.

The point here is that there is not one thing you need to do, regardless of your lifestyle, needs, or anything else. There are many methods! They are all different, they all have their own unique challenges and benefits, and they can all be toyed around with until you find the one that works for you.

And that is really what this is about—finding the thing that works. You may already have noticed that we have talked about fasting as something from Ancient Greece and the Middle Ages. You might be asking yourself, "Is this really going to work in the modern world? Can it be brought into a society that is all about smartphones, streaming television, and drone delivery services?"

The answer is a resounding YES! It not only *can* be adapted to modern needs, but it *should* be, because we have learned so much about the body since Hippocrates, and so much more about the benefits of fasting—not just that it works, but how. It would be ridiculous to try and bring some ancient, vestigial medical practice into the modern world. We want something that is going to work—and intermittent fasting is just that, with the science to prove it.

And so, without further ado, we all want to get on the path that leads to greater health, happiness, and fewer trips to the doctor.

This is the way to get that done. So, let's go.

Chapter 1:

Benefits of Intermittent

Fasting

We have already talked a little about the benefits that might accrue from intermittent fasting. We have said that it increases health and helps us lose weight—but the big picture here is actually much more expansive than that. The benefits of intermittent fasting are far-reaching and, by all accounts, may have a profound effect on our body, even down to the genetic level!

Which, yes, I recognize sounds like it is going to turn us into mutants or something. Rest assured, intermittent fasting is not what gave us the *Creature from the Black Lagoon*. But the practice does affect us on the most granular level, except in a positive way.

In which way would that be, you ask? Let us start with an article over at Healthline to get us started.

Fasting and Insulin

To begin with, fasting affects our insulin production by making it drop. At the same time, it encourages your body to dramatically increase its production of human growth hormone, or HGH, which sounds like it is going to turn us into a giant diabetic, but actually what happens is the body burns fat at a significant level (Gunnars, 2021).

Now, while this is happening, the body removes waste material from cells, which is, interestingly enough, largely deposited into your lungs and exhaled. This process of removing waste material from your cells is part of your body's repair process, which is essential for your overall health. And, lastly, you wind up with non-mutant-creating changes in gene expression, which in this case are related to longevity and protection against disease (Gunnars 2021).

Which means what, exactly? Well, during your fast, your body begins a process of fat burning, which makes you leaner. And, at the same time, it gives itself room to remove waste products from your cells and makes you better able to fight disease and live longer.

Hardly the *Creature from the Black Lagoon*, right?

But let's zero in on a couple of these points. To begin with, weight loss is a goal many, if not most, people have when they begin intermittent fasting. We have covered how the practice affects insulin production, but what is the big picture on how it affects weight loss?

Fasting and Weight Loss

Firstly, there is the obvious point that when you fast, you eat fewer meals. Fewer meals mean fewer calories. I mean, duh. So, provided you do not double up when you break your fast—i.e., eat crazy amounts more food to make up for having fasted— then you'll lose weight.

But for specifics on how insulin production and HGH affect weight loss, what happens is these processes encourage your body to break down body fat, which your body uses for energy. This means your metabolism has been increased and, voila, weight loss.

"But wait," you might ask. "Does this mean that fasting involves both taking in fewer calories *and* increasing your metabolic rate? Isn't that like tackling weight loss from two different angles?"

Great observation, dear reader. In fact, that is precisely what this means.

Here are some numbers to help drill home this point:

- With intermittent fasting, you can lose as much as 3–8% of your body weight over 3–24 weeks.

- Participants in a study lost 4–7% of their waist circumference over 6–24 weeks. This means that they lost fat specifically in the abdomen, which is the fat most associated with disease.

- A 2011 review said that intermittent fasting is less likely to decrease muscle mass than continuous calorie restriction (Gunnars 2021).

Those are insane stats. Any activity that reduces abdominal fat in particular is worth taking a second look at, since that fat causes a significant number of diseases. We are talking heart disease, liver problems, and a whole host of things you would be better off without.

With this in mind, reducing fat is not just an aesthetic choice. It is a legitimate health choice! Preventable disease is just that—preventable. And if intermittent fasting can help us reduce problematic fat, without sacrificing muscle mass (which is not just an aesthetic choice either), then it would be foolish not to at least give it our consideration.

Now, let's get back to a couple other things we discussed earlier. We mentioned that intermittent fasting encourages the body to remove cellular waste. What does this mean specifically? And in what way is it good for us?

Autophagy: What Happens to Cellular Waste?

Let's start with the basics. We all know that cells are the building blocks of life. Cells are made up of various parts, which, over time, tend to stop working or do not work quite as well. In this way, they become "junk."

Autophagy, which literally means "self-devouring," is the term for what happens when your body gets rid of the junk parts of your cells. Basically, the cell determines that some part of it is not working and chooses to discard it. This is important because if a cell does not or cannot chuck off the junk part of it, then you wind up with a whole host of health problems.

What causes autophagy is, basically, stress. And not the kind where you take on too much work or whatever—the kind where you put your cells into survival mode.

Essentially, the cell has to eat itself in order to survive, which causes it to get rid of the junk. This sounds like it is bad for the cell, but it makes the whole system function way better. Some of the proximate causes include things like calorie restriction and exercise, but also, yes, fasting. This process is important because accumulation of that cellular junk is not exactly good for you.

In fact, there are plenty of conditions that are now understood to be associated with autophagy. These include such beauties as Crohn's disease, diabetes, heart disease, Huntington's disease, kidney disease, liver disease, and even Parkinson's disease. There is also evidence that links problems with autophagy to cancer: Accumulating "junk" in the cell might screw with replication, which is what starts that process ("Autophagy," 2012).

Now, the Cleveland Clinic makes sure to note that autophagy has been described as a health trend and that there needs to be more research done to understand its benefits as a "wellness strategy" ("Autophagy," 2012). And fair enough! As we said earlier, the last thing we want to do is jump on some health bandwagon. We want proven strategies for healthy living, not some fad to get caught up in.

So, let's flag autophagy for now, but with an addendum: There are signals right now that autophagy might be an important part of a healthy living strategy. For example, it is true that defects in autophagy are linked to the diseases listed above. So, if it winds up being true that inducing autophagy is good for us and can prevent those illnesses, and fasting can induce autophagy, then we have one more reason to consider intermittent fasting as a health choice. If not, then there are plenty of other reasons aside from that to keep us going.

Fasting and Inflammation

One of those reasons would be the effects of fasting on inflammation.

Now, inflammation itself is a perfectly natural process. In fact, it is one of the ways our bodies fight disease! What happens to cause inflammation is that your body recognizes some kind of pathogen or harmful intruder and begins the healing process.

Now, there are two types of inflammation: Acute and chronic. Acute inflammation occurs when you have some sort of tissue damage, say from trauma or if a pesky microbe has snuck into your body. This can last two to six weeks and is not usually cause for concern. Chronic inflammation, however, is a different story. It can last up to several years and has a number of different causes.

For starters, maybe your body just can't get rid of whatever has gotten inside of it. There are some parasites, for example, that are super resilient to our immune responses. Continuously trying to get rid of them might cause the infected area to become chronically inflamed. You might also have some kind of autoimmune disorder that thinks that a perfectly normal part of your body is actually harmful. Or, you might have defective cells that cause this or that area to become inflamed.

Whatever the case, chronic inflammation is an indicator that something has gone wrong with the immune response. And that is not all, because chronic inflammation is also associated with a whole host of terrible diseases.

The rogues' gallery of illnesses here includes diabetes; cardiovascular diseases, including coronary heart disease and stroke; and COPD, which is the third most common cause of death in the United States. In fact, these chronic diseases are considered the most significant causes of death in the world, and upward of 60% of Americans have one of them. That number is not expected to decrease, either—if anything, it is just going to go up (Pahwa et al, 2023).

Okay, so enough of the doom and gloom already, right? Where is the silver lining?

According to experts, intermittent fasting can reduce inflammation. How it does this is by reducing what are called "monocytes" in the blood, a kind of white blood cell that causes inflammation. Fewer monocytes, less inflammation; less inflammation, less chronic inflammation as a cause of multiple preventable diseases (Berger, 2019).

The reason for this is interesting. While it might be tempting to conclude that starvation—even controlled starvation—is the cause of this reduction in monocytes, it might be that, instead, most of us are just eating too damn much. Given that constant eating is a recent phenomenon in the history of our species, its co-occurrence with chronic-inflammation-related illness is interesting. Essentially, we are over-fueling ourselves, and time-restricted eating is one way of correcting this.

One study, according to the article I have been citing here, had participants fast between noon and 3 p.m. the same day, then start fasting again at 8 p.m. that same day and not eat until 3 p.m. the next. On both days, at 3 p.m., blood was drawn, and white blood cells were tested (monocytes are a type of white blood cell). What they found was a reduction in these cells, below what would be typical for a healthy human being (Berger, 2019).

And that is not all! Obviously, this is all just preliminary, and many more studies will have to be done to confirm what has been said here. But this is an interesting signal—because if fasting can reduce monocytes, which reduces inflammation, and chronic inflammation causes multiple preventable diseases, then intermittent fasting could potentially prevent those diseases from occurring in the first place.

The State of the Research: Fasting and Longevity

Now, it should be reiterated for safety that research remains in the beginning stages. Of course, information might arise in the future that contradicts these claims.

But there is reason to be excited! What if this ancient, time-worn technique really could be used to reduce coronary heart disease, stroke, and COPD? Living without these deadly illnesses really could be as simple as selectively not eating for periods throughout the day or week.

To make matters even more interesting, there is also the science around longevity, or how long people live for.

Understanding what makes people live a long time is still in its infancy. What we do know is that several factors contribute to a long life, including environmental and social factors, but also genetics. When we look at people who have lived into their 90s, and especially people in excess of 110 years old, we find several interesting facts about them: To begin with, education and income do not seem to have an effect, which runs counter to most people's expectations ("Is Longevity Determined by Genetics?" 2022).

What they do have in common tends to be things like not smoking, not having weight problems, and dealing well with stress. On its own this might help explain some of what allows them to live so long; however, it appears as though lifestyle choices are significant for the first seven or eight decades, after which genetics becomes much more important ("Is Longevity Determined by Genetics?" 2022).

As with virtually everything else we have talked about in this chapter, our understanding of which genes make us live longer is still in its infancy. And, in fact, much of what we are finding is a bit on the confusing side. For example, people who live to be in their 90s have the same disease-causing genes as the rest of us, but supercentenarians—people in excess of 110 years of age—have genetic sequences that appear unique to them ("Is Longevity Determined by Genetics?" 2022).

But while there is still much to learn, genetics does seem to play a role in deciding who gets to live several decades past the norm. This means that the answer to the question of whether or not we can extend human life probably lies in the direction of genetics.

And do we want to extend our lives? As far back as one of our earliest stories, today known as *The Epic of Gilgamesh*, we have been thinking about what it would mean to escape death. Although *Gilgamesh* and many others are focused on immortality, which is inarguably the most extreme version of life extension, humanity has spent an awful lot of its energy on learning how to either avoid the inevitable or, at the very least, keep it at bay.

In fact, we might argue that the whole reason we have medicine in the first place is to delay the inevitable. Lord knows our ancestors had to deal with the blunt effects of nature, with all of its billions of ways to put us in the ground. Learning about how nature works is essentially the way we learn to combat it.

And look, let's be honest. Most of us, when we are asked about whether we would like to live a long time or not, wind up saying something like, "No way! Live into my 90s? Why, so I can be miserable and sick and old?"

But guess what? By the time we are 80, we will want to live to be 85. By the time we are 85, we will want to live to be 90—

and so on. So why beat around the bush? We all want to live a long life and there is no shame in it.

The good news is that intermittent fasting can help us get there.

Consider what was said earlier about people who live insanely long. Obviously not smoking helped them get there, and there are other factors too, like not drinking too much and getting enough exercise. But one of the things these people had in common is that they were not overweight. Remembering that time-restricted eating has a positive effect on weight loss, we are already on our way to living a long life.

But there is more to this: It turns out that intermittent fasting alters the expression of genes, and specifically those related to longevity.

Research is now saying that, when tested on mice, intermittent fasting has a "system-wide" effect on both body and brain. In fact, when mice who were put on time-restricted diets had their organs tested after the experiment, scientists found that upward of 70% of each mouse's genes responded to the diet (Cadogan, 2023).

One of the most affected areas was the adrenal gland, which is responsible for hormone production. Improper hormone balance has been linked to all sorts of illnesses, from diabetes through to what are called "stress disorders." Given that time-restricted eating affected something like 40% of the adrenal gland's genes, intermittent fasting might be a key factor in maintaining hormonal balance and limiting the prevalence of related disorders (Cadogan, 2023).

Maybe most interestingly, the findings stated that intermittent fasting has an effect on our circadian rhythm, which is our body's natural cycle of sleeping and waking. Disruptions of our circadian rhythms are basically the opposite of healthy and can lead to such horrible outcomes as cancer. Shift workers in particular have a heck of a time with their health for this reason, which means some of our most important jobs, from firefighters to paramedics, are by their nature unhealthy for us to perform.

Our circadian rhythm is not just limited to one part of our body, either. Every cell is on a circadian rhythm. The results of one study said that intermittent fasting helps align the circadian rhythm across the whole system, which led to improvements in the health of firefighters (Cadogan, 2023). Considering the importance of jobs like that, ensuring that firefighters can live long without being plagued by job-related cancers would be a positive outcome.

In other words, by altering our bodies on the genetic level, intermittent fasting can help reduce the likelihood of early death and perhaps also make us live longer. Although there is still much to learn about how genetics influence longevity, the fact that they seem to play a role, and that intermittent fasting appears to influence them in such a way that they are less likely to induce illness, suggests that the practice of fasting might be an integral part of increasing our longevity.

Of course—coming back to what we said about living longer before—living longer is fine and all, but when quality of life goes down the tubes, a long life is more of a prison than anything. For most of us, when we think of being elderly, we think of not just being frail, but being "not quite with it."

Dementia, in other words, is a terror most of us feel. We know it can happen. Many of us have seen it firsthand. It remains, and will always remain, a devastating horror of an illness that, given the choice, all of us would choose to avoid.

Well, guess what? It looks like fasting might help with that too!

Fasting and Dementia

Let us pause for a second here. I know this is sounding too good to be true—I do! Anything that promises to make you lose weight, live longer, be healthier, and maintain your brain health all at the same time is inherently suspect. I get it.

Which is why, before I go on with this, I want to emphasize that there is much to learn about the science of health and medicine. But what we are talking about here are various signals that fasting is connected with a slew of health benefits. What that will look like in the future—who knows? For now, though, this is all very interesting and should not be construed as some kind of snake oil, or a cure-all for everything that has ever ailed human beings.

With that in mind, let us move onto brain health!

Yes, intermittent fasting appears to have a positive effect on our brains. One of the ways it does this is by increasing the production of a protein called brain-derived neurotrophic factor. This protein is important because it encourages the growth of new neurons and synapses, and in doing so helps improve things like cognitive function. In other words, you are able to think better!

There is also a potential effect on a process called "neurogenesis," which is where new neurons are made in the region known as the hippocampus. This is the region that is responsible for our cognition, learning, and memory.

And is that all? Not on your life! Because if we return to what we said earlier about the effects intermittent fasting has on inflammation and insulin, it turns out that these processes affect the brain also. Diabetes in particular has been linked to various brain diseases, but inflammation is no better (Panuganti, 2023).

And remember our friend autophagy? Well, it is a key process in the brain as well. In fact, getting rid of cellular junk in the brain might help stave off brain disorders, including those of a neurodegenerative kind—namely, dementia and Alzheimer's disease (Panuganti, 2023). Essentially, if intermittent fasting encourages autophagy, and autophagy helps prevent dementia, then intermittent fasting might be one of the key ways we can prevent the onset of that terrible disease.

So, what does this look like altogether?

Concluding the Basics

If what these studies are saying is true, then intermittent fasting might have a whole slew of benefits. These extend through not just keeping us at a healthy weight but reducing incidences of a number of diseases of the body and the brain. And on top of that, it seems to add a spiritual dimension to the lives of those who practice it.

Is it a cure-all? Well, what is? What it is, however, is a possible key to helping us live long and healthy lives, and all at the cost of being hungry for short periods of time—on purpose.

But for how long should we stay hungry? What are some of the ways in which we can make sure we are doing this in a way that is healthy? And what are some of the benefits—and costs—of each of these methods?

Chapter 2:

Implementing Intermittent

Fasting

One of the things we find in the literature on intermittent fasting is that, in order to pull it off, you need to follow a set schedule. In other words, you do not fast whenever the moment strikes you, or at random times. You know when the fasting is going to happen and for how long, and you stick to it.

But what should that schedule look like? How long should somebody fast for at a time? These are important questions. Luckily for us, there are a bazillion different ways to do this. And one of them, I am sure, will turn out to be the right one for you.

Fasting Protocols: A Brief Glance

Maybe the easiest one, and therefore best for beginners, is to fast for 12 hours a day. This is simple, straightforward, and, yes, easy to do. You simply choose a 12-hour window in which you will not eat—say, from 8 p.m. to 8 a.m. You can consume the same number of calories as you normally would in a day, you just do it within that 12-hour window. According to some research, a 10–16-hour fast should encourage the body to burn fat by releasing ketones (Leonard, 2023).

A fast that lasts for 16 hours actually has its own name! This is called the 16:8 fast and is usually done when somebody skips breakfast every morning. The first meal of the day then is lunch. (And who has not done that from time to time?) One of the reasons somebody might be interested in this particular diet is that they have given the 12-hour one a whirl and it did not work for them, but it is also good to try for its own sake. In fact, when mice have been exposed to this particular diet, incidences of diabetes, obesity, and other illnesses dropped. And this was true even if they ate their standard number of calories in that eight-hour window (Leonard, 2023).

Next up is a fast called the 5:2 diet, which is when you fast for two consecutive days a week. Now, this does not mean consuming zero calories during that period, because that would be super dangerous. Instead, people typically consume 500–600 calories a day during their fast days.

The difficulties with this one are obvious. For those two days you are probably going to be groggy, so you will want to plan accordingly. Do you have to, for example, operate heavy machinery during that period? Are you in charge of safety at the nuclear power plant? Really think hard about whether this one is right for you before you do it.

Another downside of the 5:2 diet is that some research suggests that weight loss is no more significant using this diet than in people who use continuous calorie restriction. But luckily, as with most fasting protocols, insulin levels are affected to the point of improving. And what is more interesting, one small-scale study found that women in particular lost weight during menstruation by using this plan. They did return to their usual weight after five days of eating their usual amount, but for the study period there was a signal that this approach might work for them (Leonard, 2023).

Now maybe the most extreme form of this practice is what is known as "alternate-day fasting." This is exactly what it sounds like: Every other day, you take in no food (although some people allow for up to 500 calories). This is, as you can imagine, an effective weight-loss strategy—over a 12-week period, participants in a study lost something like 11 pounds each (Leonard, 2023). Nothing to sneeze at!

But this one is obviously a little on the challenging side. Not that it is inadvisable, especially for people who desperately need to lose weight fast and can undertake this protocol with medical supervision. The problem, of course, is that it is difficult enough that most people will stop doing it. And not just that, but most of us have to work for a living, and spending half our workdays groggy from not eating is not going to be good for our performance. This one is really something you would need to talk to your doctor about. But for some people, it might be just the solution they need.

For others, there is the standard 24-hour, one-day-a-week fast. This is exactly what it sounds like: no calories for a full 24-hour period. The side effects here would be no different than any of the others—namely, that you will be exhausted and irritable— but many practitioners have said that over time, the body adjusts, and the side effects become less intense. If you are curious about this one, it is definitely something you would be best off working your way up to. Maybe you have tried a 12-hour fast, maybe you have tried a 16-hour fast. You feel like you are ready for a big one, so you give 24 hours a spin. Some people really swear by it! If you think you are up to it, then it might be what is right for you.

And now it is onto the Warrior Diet.

If this one sounds to you like it must be for gladiators, or some ancient, barbaric version of Arnold Schwarzenegger, then you are not far off. How it works is that you eat small servings of raw fruit and vegetables at the most within a 20-hour window. The following four-hour window is when you consume the number of necessary calories to keep you going.

The trick, though, is that the four-hour window occurs at night. Adherents to this diet swear that humans are naturally nocturnal eaters and therefore eating before bed is the best time to do so.

Now, are there some problems with this? Obviously. One thing people find is that their intake of fiber tends to take a hit, which can lead to health problems (like cancer, for the record). Also, eating 2,000 calories before bed is going to be difficult to maintain for long periods. But, as with the others here, there are those who swear by it. And for the adventurous caveman warriors among us, especially those who can make sure that what they eat in that four-hour period includes all the vitamins and minerals they need to survive, this might be the kind of barbarian challenge they are looking for.

Problems and Solutions

The thing is, no matter which plan you choose, you will run into problems. As Thomas Sowell famously said, in life there are no perfect solutions, only trade-offs. So, with each of these plans there are costs and benefits, risks, and rewards.

The real question is how to maintain any of these plans once you get started. Because do not kid yourself, some of them are very challenging. So, we will need to come up with ways in which we can stick to our goals, push through the difficulties, and reap the rewards of intermittent fasting.

One of the more obvious strategies involves staying hydrated. Drink not just water, but herbal teas and other low to no calorie drinks throughout the day. You will need electrolytes, for example, so these are going to be essential (Leonard, 2023). But it is also true that you need to keep your stomach full, and you need to busy your hands and mouth with something. Making sure to drink water is a good way to cover all these bases and ensure you are on a path to success.

You are also going to want to avoid thinking about food. Which—yeah, I know, it sounds stupid. Especially since we all know that trying not to think about something only makes you think about it more. But the thing is, if you think about food, you are going to get hungry. That is just how it works.

So, what you will want to do is find ways to distract yourself. For example, you might go for a walk (although strenuous exercise while fasting is not recommended). You might take in a movie or do some menial task that needs to get done. Cleaning your apartment is not a bad idea during this time either. Basically, whatever you can do to get food off your mind, do it.

Light exercise is another way you might keep yourself occupied. Yoga, for example, would not be your worst bet. But trying to relax during fast days is a fantastic way to keep yourself centered and focused. You do not hear about Buddhist monks taking a day off eating and then trying to beat their deadlift record. Just take it easy, stay relaxed, and do not hurt yourself.

When you are eating, you will want to make sure that you are not filling yourself up with junk either. Breaking a fast does not mean going through the drive-thru and ordering 55 tacos, 55 burgers, and 150 pies. It means you need to fill up on things that are going to keep you healthy and let you get through the next fast. So, try to eat plenty of fruit, fish, lentils, and beans.

High-volume foods are also a great choice! Grapes and melons would be a couple of examples, but, in general, it is good to fill up on things that actually fill you up in order to avoid overeating. Popcorn is another great example and can commonly be found in the movie theater, the happiest place on earth.

Now, I have never been a person who is worried so much about food taste. I have a soft, British palate that my Northern Irish ancestry has gifted me, meaning I can eat boiled potatoes with no salt and not bat an eye. However, this, as I understand it, is not the norm. So, in order to maximize your enjoyment while getting in your meals, it might be wise to try seasoning and/or other methods for getting flavor into your food.

Essentially, what all of this means is that there are a bunch of different methods you can use or adapt to increase your odds of success. Some of these may work for you, others might not. There are probably tons of them I have not thought of here, meaning there are plenty more waiting to be discovered.

Considering how different we all are in physiology and psychology, no one particular method is going to work for everyone. Some of you may find you like the Warrior Diet and that drinking herbal tea and using tons of seasoning on your meals is a great way to pull that off. Others may find that fasting every other day works so long as they can stay busy on their fast days.

That is great! These are meant for mixing and matching. The whole reason there are so many options in the first place is that people have been experimenting with them, analyzing the results, and coming to a particular conclusion about how well the method works. You, of course, can do the same.

With that in mind, we have to move onto some essential caveats here.

A Few Essential Caveats

To begin with, yes, these are all going to be challenging. But if you go into any of them unprepared, you are going to be in serious trouble. For example, if you do not consume enough calories or water on your eating days, then fast the day after, it's not a good idea.

As with any strenuous activity, it is important that you go in fully prepared for what is coming. It is like going to the gym: You do not do it without taking in some carbs first, staying hydrated, and making sure you start with stretches. Doing it any other way is going to hurt you.

But maybe the most important thing to keep in mind is that intermittent fasting is not a good idea for people who are prone to eating disorders.

Recent research suggests that there might, in fact, be a strong link between the two behaviors. A study out of the University of Toronto, for example, found that women who engaged in intermittent fasting also tended to engage in associated eating disorder-related behaviors. This includes things like laxatives, vomiting, and compulsive exercise (Citroner, 2022).

Part of the reason for this might be that fasting affects our reward pathways. For someone with anxiety, this means that fasting may calm them down; the brain registers this as a positive, naturally, and then encourages the individual to do it again and again, often at more dangerous levels.

For these reasons and many more, we have to be cautious when implementing these methods. Young people, in particular, are at a high risk of developing an eating disorder, which means that, if intermittent fasting has the potential to develop into an eating disorder in itself, then young people should be particularly wary about using fasting as a means toward a healthy lifestyle.

Some of the downsides, of course, can be traced back to social media. It is well known by now that social media is effectively a scourge upon this planet, but with regards to how fasting is promoted it has shown itself yet again as a vector for spreading risky behaviors.

Getting information regarding how to fast from social media is as risky as getting anything from social media. You do not know who your sources are, what they know, what their intentions are—nothing. Considering the risks associated with fasting, it is best to consult medical professionals, especially those in, for example, dietetics. You do not want to get your information from someone who may be engaging in risky behavior in order to become a more popular internet personality.

The problem, of course, is that young people in particular do get their information from social media. And group dynamics being what they are, many of them are lulled into a pattern of risky behavior that might not be obvious to them at first.

The point here is that forewarned is forearmed. Preparation, as with anything, is the key to success. If you are young, it is best to stay away from fasting, no matter what is happening in that dreaded domain of social media. And if you are prone to eating disorders, please know that the difference between a healthy fast and one that has become a compulsive eating disorder is an easy line to cross—especially if you are burdened by that predilection to begin with.

Talk to your doctor. Do not do anything crazy. Keep your goals in mind. And talk to your doctor again.

Okay. We have got that stuff in play now. But we do not want to end on an unhappy note, so we just have one more stop to make before we can close out this chapter.

The Benefits of a Good Plan

Creating a plan is one of the best and easiest ways to ensure success. Not just in our fasting life, but in all areas—work, free time, everything. The benefits are numerous, so let us go through a few of them here.

First, creating a plan helps you find a balance in your activities. It can be easy to go all-in on something and forget about the rest of your life. For example, maybe you have started going to the gym for the first time. You feel great, and you like what is happening to your body.

Many of us have had the experience (or maybe it is just me!) where we follow that realization with, "I should just go to the gym all the time then!" Now this is understandable in the sense that we all enjoy getting the results we are looking for. And certainly, there is no shame in wanting to put in more work!

But we do live multifaceted lives, all of us. We do not just exercise, or work, or spend time with our families. We do all of those things, and we need to find a balance to keep them all afloat.

This is no different with fasting. We want to be prepared and we want to be successful, but we do not want it to take up our entire lives. Creating a schedule can help prevent us from spending our family time thinking about the fast—that has already been done and it is just waiting to be implemented.

It also helps us keep track of progress. For example, when I quit smoking years ago, it was hard getting through the first day. When I did, I looked back on it with a sense of accomplishment. Getting through two days felt even better. Then three, four.

By the time I was a month in, the idea of going back seemed almost unthinkable. I had all those days behind me. Why would I want to start from zero again? I had already come so far.

Getting through one fast is an incredible effort. And I am sure you will feel a sense of accomplishment. But when you keep to a schedule, you get to see how many you have managed to pull off and, if it is a healthy amount, you can feel a sense of pride in what you have done.

It is also, coming back to our earlier point, a good way to make sure you are not going overboard. Maybe you are feeling unwell and cannot figure out why. Having a board or a calendar to tell you that you have been hitting it too hard might be useful, so you know how to adjust and correct.

It also helps you remain accountable. When you see failures pile up, it can diminish your confidence, sure, but it can also be the kick in the ass that you need. You said you were going to do such and such a thing, and, by God, you are going to do it!

When you make the commitment to fasting and want to pull it off, coming in prepared, making sure you know what you are doing, and ensuring you have covered all the possible health-related risks that might come into play are even more important than the fast itself. Do not do anything dangerous!

With all that in mind, I think we have covered the benefits of scheduling and the importance of safety. But we have only just touched on the fasting protocols themselves!

What are the positives and negatives for each one? What are some testimonials related to them? Why might we be interested in one over another? And what are some unique challenges that might arise as a result of implementing a specific one?

Let's find out!

Chapter 3:

Popular Intermittent Fasting

Protocols

The number of individual fasting protocols is long and, I am sure, will only get longer with time. Given how popular intermittent fasting has become, it can even seem like there might be too many different types!

So, here we are going to run through which ones are the most popular, what the benefits and drawbacks are to each of them, and what unique challenges arise when implementing them. (You will notice that these were mentioned in the previous chapter, so consider this a deep dive!) The goal here is to get as much information about these things into this book as we can, but there will always be things we miss. There are different fasting protocols, safety and health issues, all kinds of things that might slip through the cracks.

Which means if you find one you are interested in and think there is more research to be done—you are probably right! Always go in with as much information as you can get a hold of. But think of this chapter as a helpful primer on what your options are.

That said, let's get started!

16:8 Fast

The first one we covered in the previous chapter was the 16:8 fast. This is where you fast for 16 hours a day and eat only during an eight-hour window. During that 16-hour fast you can consume water, coffee, and tea, provided there are no additives (sugar and cream have calories, remember). But other than that, you are calorie-free.

So how does this work? Is it something you do every day? Every week? What kinds of foods are best consumed during your eight hours to ensure the 16-hour fast doesn't totally knock you into next week?

The nice thing about this one is that you can do it at whichever frequency you are most comfortable with. For example, you might only want to do this once a week. Knock yourself out! The plan does not necessarily lend itself to a set number of repetitions. It only says how long you should fast for if and when you choose to.

One of the benefits of this type of fast, as said earlier, is that it appears to burn fat. It also affects your blood sugar and, adherents believe, increases your longevity (Streit & Amjera, 2023). That is a lot from such a straightforward procedure!

Because it is easy to implement, it is a much simpler way to accomplish your goals. As we will see with other types of fasts, it is possible to follow a much more complicated set of rules. This one is simply that, on whichever day you choose to follow it, you stay away from calories all day other than in your eight-hour food window.

Now, is there a time of day you should fast in order to get the maximum results? Is there a bad time to fast? The answer is a firm "not really." The flexibility of this fast also includes when you decide to do it during the day. For example, since most people are awake from 12 p.m. to 8 p.m., that is not a bad time to schedule your eating period. But if you prefer something earlier or later, that's fine—maybe you work the night shift and are not awake in the early afternoon. Whatever you want, whenever you want, it all works, so long as you make sure to fast for 16 hours in a row.

One of the things we want to make sure of is that when you are eating, you are getting all the nutrients you need to get you through your day. That means no chips or cookies. That is wasted space in your stomach. You want to eat things that are healthy, because if you slip in that department then you are going to be in trouble.

To begin with, you want to make sure you get lots of fruit. Apples, bananas, tomatoes, the whole slew of them. The health benefits we get from eating fruit are legion and they should absolutely be a part of your diet.

No diet is complete without vegetables, and that goes for this one as well. Make sure to eat plenty of variety in this department. That means everything from carrots and broccoli through to cucumbers and leafy greens like lettuce and kale.

Whole grains are going to be key here too. Rice and oats are perfect, which means overnight oats might be just the thing you need. But you will want to balance this out with some healthy fats, like the ones you get from avocados, and of course protein sources. That means eating fish, eggs, nuts, and seeds.

A lot of this may seem like a bit of a "Yeah, duh," but your food health is important! Fasting can take a lot out of you and you need to be strong and prepared to pull it off.

Of course, the benefits here are as we discussed earlier— namely, that you undergo weight loss, your blood sugar control becomes stronger, and you may even have increased longevity.

But there are some downsides to this one that we need to think about also.

For starters, it is likely that you will have the desire to overeat when you get off the fast. This is totally normal! But remember that doing so can lead to weight gain and digestive problems, among other things. So, go into it knowing that this desire might be strong, and have a plan in place to curb it, if possible. Maybe meal planning is your friend here!

5:2 Diet

Next up is the 5:2 diet. We will remember this as the one in which you eat regularly for five days, and then fast for two. The maximum calorie intake while fasting here is 600 calories, but many people prefer 500. Either way is up to you.

Now right off the hop, this one is harder than the previous one. Restricting yourself to such a small number of calories is hard enough to do once a week, let alone twice. This will require perseverance, control, and hard work. But if we go in with the right amount of preparation, it is totally possible!

To begin with, there is some research on this type of fast that should be of interest to us. The fine folks over at Healthline report that a study found the benefits of the 5:2 fast were not largely different from those gained through traditional dieting. However, and this is interesting, the participants were actually more likely to continue with the fast than they were with the traditional diet (Bailey, 2021).

This means that even if it lacks an advantage in the amount of weight lost, fasters are more likely to be successful in the long term because they tend to stick with the program. And considering how many people yo-yo diet, maybe this method is a way to break the cycle.

Part of the reason for this is that participants actually reported enjoying fasting more than dieting (Bailey, 2021). What exactly was more enjoyable about this program I can't say for sure, but enjoying what you do is such a necessary ingredient for success that without it, you are almost certain to fail. Consider all the awful tasks you have ever done throughout your life—maybe it is some menial job for low pay, where your boss yells at you all the time and you cannot get along with anybody else on the floor. (Not just me, I hope!) If you compare your productivity at a job like that to one where you get along with everybody, find your work meaningful, and get paid a wage you think is fair, I will bet dollars to doughnuts you were way more successful at the latter job, at least in terms of accomplishing your goals.

This is a fundamental axiom of life. Why would dieting be any different? Maybe you enjoy fasting more because it is novel, or because it feels like more of an accomplishment to withhold calories throughout the day. Who knows? Whatever the case, your enjoyment is an essential ingredient to accomplishing the task, and the participants in the study on the 5:2 diet can only corroborate this.

The downsides to this are largely the same as with all the other methods—namely, that certain people in particular should avoid this type of activity, such as those prone to eating disorders and those who can't take medication on an empty stomach. Also, anyone under 18 should be cautious about doing this.

However, with regards to benefits, it is also possible that fasting can help with enhancing your motor coordination and lowering your cholesterol. So, you take the good with the bad!

Eat Stop Eat

The last protocol we are going to look at here is the Eat Stop Eat method. This one is similar to the 5:2 method, except it is more intense. Basically, you choose one or two nonconsecutive days in a week, and you take in zero calories. Not 500, not 600—zero.

Its origins can be traced back to a fellow by the name of Pilon. This guy wrote a book called *Eat Stop Eat* in which he detailed the ins and outs of the plan. According to him, the seed for this protocol was developed when he was researching the effects of fasting while at the University of Guelph (which is in Canada, for those of you elsewhere). As he puts it, this is a nontraditional way of going through a fast, because it is intended to make you rethink your relationship to food. Specifically, things like meal timings are to be reconsidered, particularly with regards to how this is related to your overall health (Pilon, 2017).

This book is strongly recommended, by the way. There is far more in between those pages than I could possibly summarize here, but if this sounds like your kind of thing, then obtaining this book should be a priority.

Now, let's get into the details.

As we said, this diet is not complicated, at least in theory: You simply pick one or two nonconsecutive days each week to take in no calories. Those days are not the kind where you can get in a few calories at the end either. Those are full 24-hour fasts.

When you are on your off days, it's up to you as to what your eating habits look like. But as we mentioned before, what you eat during these periods is crucial. You have the option of eating trash, of course, but why not make better food choices?

Why not take in fruits and vegetables instead of McDonald's and delivery pizza? You are, after all, going to go 24 hours with no food. You should make what you eat count.

Notice, however, that a 24-hour period still means you get to eat something every day. "Wait," you say, "that doesn't make any sense!" Yes, it does, and please let me finish. Maybe you eat breakfast at 8 a.m. normally. You are up an hour before that to make sure you are ready. If you have chosen 8 a.m. as the beginning of your fast, which means it ends at 8 a.m. the next day, you are up for an hour before it starts. If you do not eat anything before your start time, you are actually extending the fast past 24 hours. You can eat at 7.30 a.m., and you are still good.

In fact, this is definitely recommended. You are about to put your body through the wringer here, so going in with a full meal to start will keep you well-fueled and capable of withstanding the day ahead.

But that is not all, of course. Hydration, as always, is going to be a crucial factor in maintaining your health through the fasting period. Hydration is recommended normally but be sure to drink tons of water while you are not eating. It will help keep you awake, for one, and it will keep your stomach relatively filled, which you will want.

With that in mind, let's go through the benefits and downsides of this specific protocol to see if it is right for you.

Weight loss is still the number one reason people are interested in fasting, but with this method, the jury is still out on whether or not it works. Not to say that it does not work, but there are currently no studies on this method specifically. Which means that throwing our hat in the ring one way or the other would be inappropriate. However, it may be the case that for some people, periodic fasting does promote weight loss. So, while we can't say for sure, there is still a chance.

That it restricts calorie intake is the most obvious signal that it would help reduce weight, since this is what it takes to lose weight in every context. The question is more about whether or not the fasting method works better than traditional calorie restriction. There are problems too with the possibility that on non-fast days, you overeat to compensate for having not eaten anything the day before.

It is the changes to our metabolic rate that might be the most promising, however. We all know that carbs are one of the fuels our body uses to make energy. Essentially, carbs are broken down into glucose, which is what is used to keep us active and alive. Once we run out of glucose, the body starts breaking down fat, which is stored energy in the body. After between 12 and 36 hours of no calorie intake, the body will have ripped through all the glucose stored in the liver and has to start burning through fat.

This is a crucial difference between fasting and traditional calorie restriction. Although research in this area is still new and therefore limited, there remains a possibility that fasting promotes improvements in body composition in a way that other diets can't (Hill, 2022).

So much for the benefits. Let's move onto the downsides.

First off, improper nutrition can for sure be a consequence of this diet. I am as guilty as anyone of thinking of food as calories, either primarily or exclusively. For example, there was a time in my early 20s where, if I was hungry, I would just eat crackers. My reasoning was that I needed food, which is energy, and so by consuming energy I would be fine.

But this obviously is not quality thinking. Food is much more than just calories! It is vitamins, it is minerals—it is a whole bunch of different things.

The problem is that this diet will almost certainly make you feel tired. The temptation would be to use the non-fast days to fill up on whatever gives you energy, instead of thinking about food as a necessary fuel source. This will only make you unhealthy as all hell. Which is why it is important to be certain that what you eat on non-fast days is going to keep you healthy and fueled; or, conversely, that you do not take in too little of what you need and wind up with unhealthy weight loss.

Another problem has to do with blood sugar. While intermittent fasting is often used as a means of improving your blood sugar, this can go the other way also. Diabetics in particular would be well-advised to rethink going down this route, as a fast day could make their blood sugar drop to alarming levels. Also, if you are taking a medication that lowers your blood sugar, you will have to adjust it on fast days to make sure you are not entering dangerous territory.

And what about hormone changes? While there remains a dearth of research on this subject, some early findings point to hormonal changes having perhaps a positive effect on women and a negative one on men, specifically with regards to fertility. This has to do with how fasting affects testosterone levels and for this reason it is not advisable for women who are breastfeeding or who are trying to conceive. However, women with polycystic ovary syndrome might benefit in some fashion from the protocol (Hill, 2022).

Lastly, we will have to go over some of the psychological effects that come with fasting. We have talked about how fasting can promote or be symptomatic of eating disorders, but there are other things to consider also. For example—and anyone who's ever had to skip even a couple of meals can attest to this—fasting might make you irritable. If you have to work with others, and know you have a tendency to get hangry, then maybe give this method a second thought.

But on top of that, it might actually lower your libido. Again, research on this is scant, but let's think about this for a second. We can't produce an adequate quantity of hormones even for sleeping when we do not have enough calories. So, how are we going to produce the hormones required to promote sexual arousal—or orgasm?

Considering how much of our romantic lives are dependent on maintaining a healthy sexual attraction to one another, will fasting have a negative impact on our marriages? If we are not married, what will a low libido do to our self-esteem? Is it worth taking a risk, or is there another method that might be better for us than fasting?

These are things to think about. And they might not apply to everybody! Every one of us is different, and not just in some motivational poster-like fashion either. Our bodies are complicated. How one of these protocols affects any one of us is, at this point, pretty well a crapshoot. So be careful but remember that you might not be affected to the same degree as someone else.

Plus, the psychological effects are not all bad. In fact, a study conducted in 2016 found that women who accomplished a fast felt more pride and a greater degree of self-control than they had at the start of the fast (Hill, 2022). If that is something you are looking for, then maybe, after you speak with your doctor, this might be the method for you.

Testimonials

Now with regard to testimonials, these are going to be important, I think, because when we are choosing which plan to follow, or whether to get started in the first place, we want to rely on real-world experience.

So, the first testimonial we are going to look at comes from a woman named Janice (Janice, 2019). She writes at the website *Salads4Lunch*, where she documents her experience with health and weight loss, often taking up a particular challenge and posting not just her results, but also her thoughts on how things went. For example, she ran four times a week for three months and wrote about that experience, even confessing when she fell off the wagon.

According to her, she tried intermittent fasting because she was feeling desperate. She had gained 30 lbs. in two years and felt like she was not being discerning enough with her eating choices. Desperation became a motivator to give a fasting program a shot, and so she took it up.

The protocol she chose was the 16:8 method. In the beginning, she said it was quite a challenge. She has kids who play hockey, and the french fries at the arena were almost too tempting to pass up.

One thing she realized, however, was that the fast (which started after 6 p.m.) gave her a new understanding of why she ate the way she did in the first place. For example, although she used to snack during the evenings, it was not because she was hungry. Turns out she was actually just bored.

A lot of us will probably be familiar with that. Food becomes something to do, basically. We watch TV and we want something to do with our hands. So, we grab a bag of chips to keep ourselves occupied. But drinking water will actually perform the same task. Or, if you like, a fidget spinner. (Do people still use those or am I showing my age?)

As for results, Janice says that in one month she lost over 7 lbs. She says it was not a difficult plan to implement because the structure of it was simple, as opposed to certain other fad diets she has tried that have been complicated. She said 16:8 led to her snacking less, which explained, she figures, the weight loss. And it was enjoyable to carry out.

Meanwhile, Jonathan Adrian, MD, tried the 5:2 fast and reported on it at *The Medium* (Adrian, 2019). As he notes, doing it throughout November meant he had eight fasting days during that month. As far as his food intake during the fast days, he tended to have hot tea with some milk in the morning, a tiny portion of chicken soup in the afternoon, and then from there apples and watermelon.

One of the things he said he learned during his fasts was that while his stomach complained about the lack of food, his brain was doing most of the "shouting." Your body of course goes into a kind of starvation mode during these periods, but he found that if he plowed through them, his brain would usually quiet down after a period.

He also says he worked out during his fast days (which, it should be noted, is not advisable). These workouts burned about 400 calories for him each day, which means on his fast days he was going into a serious deficit. Because of this, however, he was able to lose 6.6 lbs. over the course of the month.

But more than losing the weight, he says, it was changing how he thought about food that was most significant. Much like the religious ascetics who have used fasting for thousands of years, a change of consciousness was the most notable consequence of fasting for him; in this instance, he found he had more of an appreciation for food.

This makes sense, right? Too much of anything makes you take it for granted. Adrian mentions that people with tons of money tend to have this problem, just as people with plenty of books do as well. Taking away something you have a lot of can only make you appreciate it more.

As for downsides, he says he did notice that the episodes of brain fog were significant. Anyone who has gone without food for a period will be familiar with this—it is why they tell you to eat a good meal before your exams. Without calories, your brain turns to mush, and you can't think straight.

Do you have to do a lot of mental work at your job? Maybe this is something to think about. Is it possible that having episodes of brain fog will make you a liability? What if you operate heavy machinery, like a crane?

This is why, as Adrian says, there are other ways to lose weight and become more mindful of your eating habits, or of food in general, that might be more advisable. Some of us just flat-out cannot afford to go through a period where our brains are not working.

As we have said before, it is important to have all the information we need at our disposal. This is about making an informed decision, after all! So yes, for Adrian, the fasting plus exercise helped him lose 6.6 lbs. in a month. Which is great! But keep in mind that, as with anything, there are trade-offs. Just make sure this is the right choice for you and that your doctor has signed off on it.

Part of making sure you are doing this in a healthy way is by planning your meals during non-fast days. Nutrition is important—maybe the most important thing of all! It is what keeps us moving, lets us think, and keeps us, ideally, from an early grave.

But if we are going to make a proper meal plan, we are going to have to learn not just about nutrition, but also about what to eat during our fasts, how to reintroduce food when we break the fast—and lots of other things.

So, with that in mind, let's get to talking about the food itself and what to do with it.

Chapter 4:

Meal Planning and Eating

Strategies

As we have said before, figuring out what you are going to eat on non-fast days is more important than for people who are not fasting at all. But just as important is knowing what to eat when you are fasting—assuming your protocol allows for such a thing.

In this chapter, we are going to cover a few things, all of them related to eating. We are going to figure out which foods to eat during and after fasting, how to plan meals, and what to do when you break your fast. In other words, this is going to be all about nutrition. So, buckle up and pay attention because this is an important one!

Eating and Drinking During a Fast

Regarding what you can eat while fasting, you will want to make sure you understand your protocol first off. If your protocol allows for 500–600 calories during fast days, great! But remember that some of the more intense ones do not allow any calories at all. So, brush up on that first.

In any case, you will want to make sure you drink tons of water. It does not have an enzymic effect (which means it does not break your fast) and is super good at getting rid of hunger pangs. Since it fills you up, your stomach is less likely to scream at you when you are not putting solid food into it.

Overall, you should aim to drink between one and three liters of water throughout the day, but you can decide whether sparkling or flat water works better for you. (Sparkling would be my choice, but who's asking?!) Also do not forget that you can throw in some lemon or berries, or even a cold tea infusion. The flavor helps mask the fact that it is just water.

Tea is also a good call for drinking while on a fast. The non-caffeinated variety can be drunk in whatever quantity you choose, even if that includes a quantity some would consider "copious." Since the lack of calories during a fast will make you feel cold too, tea might be a good idea if you need to be warmed up.

A couple of problems you might run into: Many of us like to put things in our tea, but since most of that includes sugar and milk, you are going to have to stay away from those. (They both have calories, obviously.) But the other thing to think of is that tea has tannins, which might make you nauseous on an empty stomach. All that means is that some teas are going to work really well for you and others are not. Shopping around is not a terrible idea.

Now, I know we are all hoping that we can drink coffee on a fast. Because, really, life without coffee is a miserable, empty black hole. And the good news is that we can! The only downside, of course, is that we cannot put anything in it. But if you are like me and prefer it black, then nothing is really going to change. In fact, research has shown that caffeine increases your metabolism, which might make it a perfect complementary substance on a fast, given what our goals are (Lett, 2021).

For downsides, though, there are a couple of obvious ones. Anyone who has ever drunk coffee on an empty stomach knows that there are all kinds of issues that come with this. For starters, it can make you feel nauseous and give you an upset stomach, which is no fun. But without food to absorb it, the caffeine kicks in that much harder. This means, if you are prone to anxiety or jitters from caffeine intake, this is going to be a problem for you.

Luckily for us, there is a type of coffee known as "bulletproof coffee," which we are going to explore here. This is a bit of a controversial addition because some people argue that drinking it breaks your fast. This is because the coffee contains a number of fats, including butter and coconut oil. Going all-in on this, by adding a boatload of fats to your coffee, can for sure count as breaking a fast, for obvious reasons.

The thing is, though, you can obviously limit the amount of butter and coconut oil you put in. Doing so will make sure you do not go over your calorie limit for the fast. And if you are a fan of keto—which frankly seems to be dying out, but time will tell—then the fats do not count anyway. Either way, limit the amount of butter you put in your coffee, and you should be fine.

Now onto apple cider vinegar—yes, *that* apple cider vinegar! One thing we know about it is that it is bursting at the seams with health benefits. For example, it affects your gut biome in such a way that it promotes its health, helps with digestion, and makes you feel full. It is also, by the way, mostly water and probiotics, which means it is not calorie-dense enough to count against your fast.

Additionally, because it makes you feel satiated, apple cider vinegar will help with those moments when the hunger begins to take over. All you need to do is toss a couple of drops into your water and you are off to the races.

Another product we can use during our fast—for those of us who are not veggie—is bone broth. First off, it is filled with minerals. But it also helps replenish your electrolytes, which you are going to be shedding through your fast. (Think of it like a healthier version of Gatorade!) It is also a good source of collagen, which will help with your stomach health—essential when you are not putting solid food into it for a whole day.

Now, it is possible that bone broth can cause a spike in your insulin levels that might, technically, break your fast. But let us be realistic here. Every diet is on a kind of spectrum, right? On the one hand we have a much more relaxed version of the diet, and on the other a much more extreme version. Thinking about whether or not bone broth will spike your insulin levels and technically break your fast is definitely extreme behavior.

Also, keep in mind that extreme behavior like this can lead to eating disorders. And we really, really do not want that! So, if you hear claims like this, that you should stay away from bone broth for the reasons listed above, my advice would be to just tune it out. You need to make sure you are comfortable and get through your day with the calories you have decided you can take in, and if bone broth helps, then why not?

Salt too is going to be a godsend, considering the electrolyte loss you are about to experience. This means you are going to be hungry and thirsty and will probably get a dry mouth. All you need to do is just dab a little salt on your tongue—not too much—and it should help with those effects.

I do not think I need to tell you not to mix the salt in with your water—because that is disgusting.

Last up on our list, we are going to talk about sweeteners. Now obviously sugar is a no-go here. But many of us have encountered the proliferation of non-sugar sweeteners over the last several years, including the ever-popular stevia. These are great because they will not cause your insulin to spike and will not toss useless calories into your day.

You can put these in your tea or coffee. Theoretically, you could even put them in your water, along with a shot of lemon. Some of you will probably have a dozen or more uses for sweeteners, given the parameters here, which is great! Be creative, make yourself comfortable, and get through your day. However you do that is up to you.

A Preliminary on Supplements

Now one area you might not think about when you are fasting is whether or not supplements break your fast, and, if so, which ones are safe to take during these periods. So, we are going to run through a few that you should not take and ones you should.

First up we have gummy vitamins. Setting aside the fact that these are for children, and you should be taking regular vitamins like an adult, they contain sugar and fat that might affect your insulin levels. If autophagy is the goal here, then the gummy vitamins might not be your best bet.

Also, seriously—just take a regular vitamin.

You should also avoid branched-chain amino acids (BCAAs). For those of you who do not know what these are, you buy them in a powder form and stir the powder into your water. They are supposed to be good for muscle growth and soreness after a workout, but also cause insulin spikes. For that reason, they are best left aside.

Speaking of workouts, protein powder is not going to be our friend here either. Alas, since it has calories, your body is not going to register that it is fasting and the whole project is kaput.

Which is too bad! Because the temptation obviously would be to use it to fill your stomach and give you an energy boost. But it just will not work and so must be left out of your fasting diet.

Meanwhile, regarding which supplements you can take during a fast, we do, fortunately, have a number of options.

First off, regular adult multivitamins. The kind you should be taking instead of gummies because you are a grown-up. Now, some multivitamins will have sugar and other additives in them—so make sure to check your labels! You want to make sure you do not toss a pill down your gullet that ruins the whole fast for you. But a multivitamin that does not ruin your fast is going to be essential to staying healthy.

Fish or algae oil are fine too! Neither of them contains enough calories to wreck your fast, provided you take them in reasonable doses. This is again something you should be checking your labels for. But considering the benefits of these types of oils, it might be wise to consider making them a part of your fasting diet.

Also, if multivitamins are not your thing (for whatever reason), then you might consider taking individual micronutrients. Just be conscious here that some vitamins are fat soluble and require you to eat food to process them. But others, such as potassium, are worth thinking about.

And although protein powder is a no-go, creatine is perfectly fine! It has no calories, which is a bonus, and does not seem to affect your insulin response. You can also take pure collagen, which might have a slight effect on autophagy, but if you are going for ketosis then this is not going to get in the way of that.

Lastly for this list, pre- and probiotics are worth considering. They do not have calories and they are good for you.

Breaking a Fast: What to Eat

Next up we are going to go through some foods you can use to break your fast. The reason we need to go over this is that, for most of us, breaking our fast means scarfing down as many calories as possible to make up for what we did the day before. This, as you can imagine, is not healthy. And so, we need to get the basics down as far as how to do it, and what to do it with.

To begin with, the best move for coming out of a fast is not to hammer back a big breakfast. Take it slow! You might even consider introducing small amounts of food at the end of your fast, just to prepare yourself for getting out of it. Your digestive system does not need a kick in the pants.

Some foods too are harder to digest than others. Anything that is high in sugar or fat is going to make you feel all gassy and uncomfortable. Big ol' greasy cheeseburgers and cake or pie— even nuts and seeds—might make you feel like rubbish.

What you will want to do is get a hold of nutrient-dense foods, ideally with some protein. This is good advice anyway, but here it is going to be a real lifesaver. With that in mind, there are some foods you may want to consider more than others, and this here is a handy list to get you started.

First up—smoothies. Who the heck doesn't love smoothies? Although they have less fiber than raw fruits and vegetables, they have tons of water, and they are super nutrient heavy. You can make them out of all kinds of things, mix things up, try new flavors—the sky's the limit. I would recommend a smoothie first thing in the morning when you break your fast.

How about dried fruits? These are what they use in Saudi Arabia to break fasts, and they work because dried fruits are jam-packed with nutrients. Apricots are a staple, but dates are fantastic too. Definitely think about using these the next morning.

Soups are, of course, a staple food almost everywhere. Everybody likes soup. I have never met a person who did not, and I do not think I ever will. Obviously, the possibilities are endless here, and you can make them easily at home with broth and vegetables you get at the grocery store.

What you will want to do here is make sure you get or make a soup that has plenty of protein, plus carbs that are not going to run havoc on your digestive system. Lentils and tofu are a good bet. Just try and be gentle when it comes to adding high-fiber sources, as this might make you feel overstuffed.

Vegetables themselves are—well, let's be honest, if you go a day without eating a healthy number of vegetables, you are not doing yourself any favors. But in terms of using them to break a fast specifically, the starchy ones like potatoes (or sweet potatoes, even better) can be a great way to come out the back end of a fast.

Fermented foods like yogurt are also worth thinking about. And if you are into avocados or some other healthy source of fat, give them a try.

All of this is to say, you have just come through a challenging activity, fasting, and you will want to be gentle on yourself coming out the other side. Your body does not need to be clobbered by something that is going to make you feel like junk, but also—and maybe more importantly—you want to make sure that you are filling up on healthy foods anyway. Loading yourself up with empty carbs is not going to do you a net positive.

Once you have reintroduced food into your system, however, you can start eating normally again—in case you thought this "go easy on yourself" diet was going to be an all-day affair.

Which does not mean overeating! I can't stress this enough! Your daily caloric intake should be the same as it is any other normal day when you come off the fast. Overeating will undo whatever you did while fasting and it is going to make you sick.

Eat clean, eat healthy, treat yourself well.

Meal Planning

A good chunk of your success is going to be dependent on meal planning. Many of us have heard about this—in fact, it might be the only diet-related subject more ubiquitous than intermittent fasting! But for how much we talk about it, few of us ever try it, and even fewer know how to do it. And considering that breaking a fast is going to be accompanied by the temptation to eat garbage, it is important that we incorporate this into our program. So, let's run through some of the basics here.

First off, yes, starting a meal plan regimen can feel a bit overwhelming. Most of us are not used to it, to begin with, and without knowing how to do it and what to expect, it can seem as though you have too many possibilities to choose from.

With that in mind, it is best to just start small! You do not have to plan every single snack and meal for your whole week right off the hop. You can plan a few of them, get your toes wet, and then add more as you get used to it.

Whether you are just starting out or you are more experienced, the big thing you will want to consider is how to make sure every food group is represented. By now we all know that you need fruits and vegetables, whole grains, and healthy fats, along with protein. Where you get these from is going to be based on your personal preference, but you will want to make sure you hit every one of these when planning your meals.

Also, if you are using recipes, you should be able to see if any of these food groups have been overlooked by looking at the ingredients. If anything has been neglected, you can adapt and fill in the blank spots.

Having an organized kitchen space is going to help also! There is nothing more frustrating than making meals for the week only to realize you do not know where some key ingredient is. Knowing where to find everything right away cuts down on time, which makes the whole process less frustrating.

Now, you might ask, is there a preferred method for making sure your kitchen is organized? The answer is, "not really." It is just a matter of making sure you know where everything is and can get it quickly. However you do that is up to you!

One thing you will want to make sure you have space for, however, is storage containers. You've probably seen the plastic Tupperware kind, or the glass ones with the resealable plastic lids. Whichever you prefer, you will want enough of them to store all of your meals in the fridge, which means making sure you have enough room to keep them there.

The reason you want these things is probably obvious, but just in case it is not: You really, really do not want to make food for the week and then find out on Wednesday it has all gone bad on you. That means you either have to start from scratch, or you get discouraged, throw in the towel, and just eat whatever. Neither of those is where we want to be.

When buying these containers, you will want to think ahead to what you will be using them for specifically. "Storing food," you might say, with a roll of your eyes. And yes, sure, but I mean, are you going to be microwaving anything? Putting things in the freezer? (Not such a simple question now, is it?) For example, plastic containers are no good for the microwave, so you will probably want glass ones. Also, the glass ones are better for the environment, if that is your thing. So, think ahead, make sure you get the right kind, and there you go.

In addition to this, you are going to want a well-stocked pantry. Certain foods and ingredients are staples and having them on hand will make this whole process way smoother. So, for starters, let's say it is good to have rice, beans, canned olives and/or tomatoes, olive oil, and peanut butter. Just to start! If you can think of any more, go for it. But keep enough of these on hand that you really only have to worry about grabbing fresh things with any degree of regularity (Hill, 2020).

Now, with regards to how much time should go into the actual planning portion, you really should only need about 10–15 minutes a week to plan (Hill, 2020). That does not mean it will take that long to actually prepare your meals, but planning is not, to be perfectly honest, that big a deal.

The good news is, there are a whole bunch of recipes all over the place, especially to do with things that can be made in huge batches, that will help you pull this off. Shop around, see if you find something you like.

Myself, I tend to get stuck on one type of meal and then eat the bejesus out of it for months and months at a time. But maybe you like to mix things up! Go bananas. Do whatever works best for you.

But seriously, do not overthink it. Grab some recipes you need for the week and then start cooking. Easy peasy!

Eating Clean

The meals themselves should be what we have already referred to as "clean." Now, this is a word that gets tossed around a lot in nutrition. But here we are going to get down to some of the nuts and bolts of it, which foods to eat, and whatever else you will need to know.

"Clean eating" basically just means not eating junk. Staying away from processed foods, candy, snacks, that sort of thing. You are sticking with the basics!

But what are the basics?

Obviously, fruits and vegetables are going to be big on this list. Any diet that tells you to restrict either of these is mistaken about what healthy eating is—and I say that without qualifications. Any and all diets should include lots of these, which are maybe the most crucial sources of nutrients and minerals in the whole of the human diet.

Breads also are a big portion of our diets. But here, instead of going for the white bread or the pale-as-hell burger buns, grab the whole-grain variety. This goes for pasta and anything else in the bread family. Remember, there are a lot of breads and bread-like products that are not as good for us as plain old whole grain. And if we are eating clean, it is a must-have.

You will also want to go easy on the meat. That does not mean cutting it out completely, by the way. But it does mean that too much meat, especially red meat, can have unwanted consequences for our diets. One rule of thumb to think about is that meat should not be the meal—it should be the side. The salad is the meal.

Processed foods, foods with tons of sugar and salt—all of these are going to get thrown by the wayside here. The total amount of time a faster is eating is less than the average person. That means every meal counts and you should take advantage of the time you have to eat as healthily as possible.

Now, all of this nutritional information is certainly not exclusive to the fasting diet. This is how to eat as healthily as possible no matter what! In the West, our diets tend to be 90% utter trash and many of our health problems are a direct result of this. Choosing to eat clean, paying attention to our nutritional intake—these are things that will only help us live longer and happier lives, with fewer instances of disease.

But of course, that is not all! There is so much more to learn with regards to nutrition. And nutrition science in general is all but brand new. New discoveries will be made all the time. And that means, as we learn more, we have a lot more adapting to do before we get the science of eating right down pat.

All this to say: You are going to be putting your body under stress when you are fasting. But the goal is to be healthy, right? We have already talked about our goals, that we want to lose weight, feel stronger, and have some control over our relationship with food.

Fasting alone will not get you there. You need to think about how best to eat right, and part of that comes down to planning meals so you are not tempted to throw in the towel and eat something you will wish you had not.

In other words, do not leave your health to chance! Take it by the reins. Achieve your goals. You are the only one who can get you there, and you are more than capable of making this happen.

Chapter 5:

Supplementing Intermittent

Fasting

Our body needs vitamins, minerals, and other types of nutrients in order to function. Most of the time we get all of this from eating. But in addition to this, we have products such as vitamin and mineral supplements, which normally can be found in a drug or grocery store.

The crucial thing to keep in mind is that there is a difference between taking in vitamins through food and through supplements. This difference is, in fact, so vast that we can't substitute healthy dietary choices for a vitamin regimen (Ravindran, 2022).

For this reason, supplements are mostly useful for people who have nutritional deficiencies or other illnesses. For us regular folk, most of our food is fortified with the kinds of materials we could be getting from supplements. (This is one of the healthy by-products of GMO farming!) You can imagine, then, that much of the research around supplement use points to, at the very best, an ambiguous relationship between supplements and our health (Ravindran, 2022).

But why is this the case? Well, for one reason, many food and drug companies test their products on animals exclusively. In other words, the trials never include human test subjects. So, while mice have been useful in extrapolating test results from, there is not a one-to-one relationship between how drugs and other products affect mice and how they affect humans.

What this means is that you are likely to run into some claims about the benefits of supplement intake that, frankly, just ain't so. A list of which supplements are useful for which conditions goes beyond the scope of our book here but suffice it to say that some are useful in promoting health in certain areas in certain people, and some are just snake oil.

That being said, it is not the case that supplements are without benefit. And since we are talking about how to keep our bodies healthy while entering and exiting periods of fasting, then supplements will be important in making sure we do not fall off a nutritional cliff.

In fact, some supplements might even help us burn fat! Which is perfect, considering that is our goal here. So, let's go through a few of them, looking at which ones to take, which ones to avoid, and, above all, why.

Taking Supplements on an Empty Stomach

As we said before, one of the things to keep in mind is that some supplements are not meant to be taken on an empty stomach. Those, maybe above all, should be avoided. Some supplements, however, either are meant to be taken on an empty stomach or can be without making you feel like rubbish. Which ones are those?

We talked about creatine already, but it is worth mentioning again. Especially if, for God knows what reason, we are crazy enough to want to work out while we are fasting, then creatine is certainly better than the omnipresent protein powder. It does not have calories, for one, and does not seem to have any effect on insulin levels (Bulletproof Staff, 2020).

The benefits of creatine are legion, which accounts for its popularity. In the most basic terms, creatine's effects are largely on the muscles, where it helps create energy, which helps you perform at your peak during a workout.

More than that, it also helps with recovery after a workout, increases your sprinting ability, and helps with brain function. And that part about brain function is key because there are signs creatine may help prevent Parkinson's, which is caused by dopamine deficits in the brain (Mawer, 2019).

All in all, creatine is not only good for you, but it might be an important addition to your fasting diet. And if exercising helps keep your mind off the lack of calories, then this will help you from getting hurt after doing so. Give it a shot!

And what about electrolytes? The trick here is that many drinks that help replenish electrolytes, or powders or however else we get them, contain sugar. And usually a lot, too. Gatorade, for example, might be great after working out (or for hangovers), but it is sugary, which means calories. Check the nutritional facts on whichever product you want to use, but if you find one without calories, it will be your friend during these trying times.

Now, I know what you are thinking: "What about L-tyrosine?" Just kidding, I know most of you are not thinking that. Who ever heard of L-tyrosine anyway?

Well, check this out. L-tyrosine is an amino acid that has some really positive effects on the brain (so sayeth the research). Essentially, it is the thing that lets your brain make dopamine, norepinephrine, and adrenaline. Altogether, that is what makes you feel good and gives you energy (Brooks, 2023).

Taken as a supplement, it might help alleviate symptoms of low mood. Not, it should be noted, that it has an effect on depressive disorders. It is not an antidepressant. It can, however, help ease your body's stress response (Brooks, 2023). Which, if we are fasting, might be something we want to consider, since fasting is by its nature stressful.

The question then of whether or not we can take it during a fast is, you guessed it, a resounding yes. In fact, it is not only supposed to be taken on an empty stomach, but in low doses is not going to break your fast.

As for pro- and prebiotics, I understand they are best taken together, and that, yes, you can take them on a fast. You will want to check out the nutrition labels on them, but if they are without calories, then you are good to go.

About probiotics: We have heard a lot of talk about the importance of a healthy gut, which in large part comes down to the levels of bacteria in there. These bacteria need to be in balance, but that balance can get thrown off by all kinds of things, including our eating habits. Not having a healthy gut can lead to problems with our immune system, as well as our general intestinal health.

But while most of what we hear about probiotics has to do with foods like yogurt or kombucha, there are also probiotic supplements we can take. And different kinds, too, each of which has its own strengths and weaknesses.

Much more information can be found on which brands do what, but I thought I would take a second to plug a few here that might be of help to you. Of course, there are a gazillion more kinds on the market, but these are some of my favorites.

For example, the well-known brand Culturelle is a great all-around probiotic supplement. It has a high colony-forming unit

(CFU) count, which the company guarantees stays viable up to the expiry date. And it does not need to be refrigerated.

If you are on a budget, however, there is always Jarrow Formulas Jarro-Dophilus EPS. This mouthful of a name might appear discouraging, but do not let it fool you. It is third-party tested to ensure potency, and, although you have to take two of them a day, they work.

For weight loss specifically, we have a particularly expensive one, but one that is worth our consideration. This is the Garden of Life brand, which, in addition to helping with weight loss, is also non-GMO certified and gluten-free, if you are into either of those things.

How does it help with weight loss, though? Well, people who are obese tend to have a bacterial imbalance in their gut. Not only might this lead to them being hungrier, but it might also result in their body storing more energy as fat than usual. Taking a probiotic like this one might help with that problem.

With all this in mind, it is worth thinking about adding probiotics into your diet, especially if you are fasting for weight loss. There are a whole bunch of other brands you can consider in addition to these but overall, they seem like an important, integral part of a healthy diet.

As for prebiotics, some of the benefits of these supplements include increasing mineral absorption and reducing the symptoms of allergic asthma. That they help with mineral absorption might be key for us, though, since we are going to be taking mineral supplements and want them to be as effective as possible.

Prebiotics also have an altering effect on gut microbiota. As we said earlier, problems with our gut biome are responsible for all sorts of shenanigans. Getting that to a healthy level, then, has myriad positive effects on us, and so should be a part of our healthy lifestyle.

Turmeric is also of help! An interesting thing about this one is that it is used in a lot of South Asian cuisine, so many of us will already be familiar with it. But there are health benefits to it in addition to tasting great, and it can conveniently be taken in ground form.

One of the most notable effects of turmeric is that it helps reduce inflammation. But one of the substances in it, called curcumin, may also protect against rheumatoid arthritis, cardiovascular disease, dementia, and even some cancers. Now it should be noted that more research needs to be done, so these conclusions are tentative. But it seems promising enough that taking ground turmeric in the morning may be advisable (Bishop et al., 2018).

Lastly, as for the water-soluble ones, vitamin C is fine on an empty stomach, and you will probably want to take some while fasting. Vitamin B, however, is a different story. Some people need a full stomach to take this, or else they will get all nauseous. If you are one of those people, then you will want to wait until the next morning to take it.

Basically, the rule here is that you want to check your labels. I mean, always check your labels anyway. But here it is extra important, because you have a goal, which is fasting, and you do not want to accidentally break your fast and ruin a whole day's effort just because you took the wrong vitamin, of all things.

So much for which vitamins to take on an empty stomach. What about the ones you should take with food? And what about ones that will break your fast, and so should be taken on your non-fast days?

Taking Supplements with Food

For chromium and vanadium fans out there, we have got some bad news for you. These supplements will lower your insulin to dangerous levels while you are on a fast. Hypoglycemia is the result, which can be an enormous pain at the low end and cause significant problems in the worst-case scenario. If you are into either of these, they should be taken when you break your fast, but, again, never during it.

Meanwhile, iodine needs to be taken with food, and magnesium will make you nauseous on an empty stomach. Also, if you are into zinc and copper, which are normally taken together, you'll want to take them with food.

Good old vitamin D is another one. We know this popularly as the sunlight vitamin because to synthesize it, we have to have access to the sun. People in cold countries or who spend a lot of time indoors are at a particular risk for deficiency. Which means Swedish writers and Canadian miners are probably super sick all the time.

Also, for the record, people with darker skin tones are at a risk of deficiency. Melanin apparently slows down the process of synthesizing vitamin D. The more you know!

One of the uses of vitamin D in our bodies is to create healthy bones, which has been known for some time. But we are actually learning a lot more about it as time goes on and finding that it has a bunch of different uses. For example, it appears as though people with low vitamin D are at a greater risk of developing a weak immune system, and might be prone to depression (Bishop et al., 2018).

And that is not all! A 2018 study found that vitamin D may help in preventing multiple sclerosis—or, at least, that people with vitamin D deficiencies are at a greater risk of developing the disease (Devje, 2023).

That goes too for respiratory health problems, including flu and COVID-19. Both of these illnesses are likely to be more severe in people with vitamin D deficiencies, so taking it might help reduce your risk of severe respiratory infection (Devje, 2023).

Crucial for us also is that vitamin D might help with weight loss. In fact, more than one study has found that taking vitamin D in addition to following a healthy diet actually made people lose more weight than the placebo group (Devje, 2023).

And the good news is, it's both cheap and accessible. So, considering that we are on a plan here to lose weight, stay healthy, and feel good about ourselves, vitamin D seems to be an almost perfect fit for us.

The only downside is that it is fat-soluble, so you'll want to take it on a non-fast day. But you should absolutely consider doing that.

Many of the others we have already covered, but it bears repeating: Fat-soluble vitamins need to be taken with food, and gummy vitamins have too much sugar in them for a proper fast. As usual, it's a simple matter of checking labels, or doing a quick Google search to figure out which ones are acceptable. (Alas, listing every vitamin and mineral available is beyond the scope of this book—and would make for an unbearably boring read!)

Now there are others too, but the ones we have covered here are a good start for us in terms of which supplements we should be taking. With them, we can make sure our mood is elevated or stable, and that problems with our gut are not making us sick. And considering that we are going whole days without putting food in there, the chance that our gut biome is going to be altered negatively is increased more than normal.

Which brings us to the main event here, folks. What have we learned about the importance of supplements—and should we take them as part of intermittent fasting?

The Verdict on Supplements

As with most things that are not the law of gravity, what we know is in a constant state of flux. The classic case here is eggs, the one food where our knowledge of its healthiness seems to always be at arm's length. One minute we should eat them, the next we shouldn't. Then we should only eat three. Then if we have ever eaten an egg, we are sure to die of cancer or cholesterol problems.

Supplements are no different. There is some research saying that we should take them, and lots saying they are snake oil. This changes depending on which supplement we are talking about too. One supplement might have health advantages where another is no better than water.

Which means that, as with everything diet-related, it's a choice you have to make. If you are going to take them, you want to make sure not only that they work, but also that they do the exact thing that you need them to. For example, taking iron pills when you are not vegetarian or anemic—what is the point? Save them for someone who needs them.

Keeping yourself healthy is important. Some of the supplements we have talked about in this chapter will help us get there and others will not. Forewarned is forearmed, knowledge is power, yada yada. Just do not believe the ones that promise you the world; take those that we have said here will help you along, do a bunch of research, and, with any luck, supplements might be just the thing for you.

Now that is covered, I think we are ready to get into some more advanced topics. So, for those of you out there who are athletes, interested in mental health, and all-around interested in high-level stuff, let's move on!

Chapter 6:

Advanced Topics

Now that we have covered the basics, let's get into some of the deeper stuff. We know that there are different types of fasts, that it's important to develop and maintain a schedule, and that nutrition, perhaps with supplements, is one of the keys to keeping yourself healthy and reaching your goals.

But there are some extenuating circumstances too, no? For example, what about athletes? Given the types of feats required of them, will fasting help or hinder them in getting to where they want?

What about the role that biological sex plays? Men and women have different bodies, and those bodies have unique concerns. Whether because of hormone levels or susceptibility to certain types of disease, men and women have to think about their health in subtly distinct ways. Does fasting affect women in ways that it doesn't affect men? How? In what ways?

And lastly, what about mental health? Considering that brain function plays such a large role in mental health, and brain function is in large part because of nutrition, will it help alleviate, or create, symptoms of mental health problems? Should people with mood disorders stay away from fasting?

Fasting for Athletes

Starting with athletics: Different sports have different nutritional requirements. That might sound silly but consider the difference between baseball and bodybuilding.

Baseball is, as George Carlin once said, a pastoral sport. It's exciting, to be sure, but it's also a nice sport. Most of the time players are not active, and what is required of them tends to be short bursts of energy, either by throwing the ball quickly or a great distance, sprinting, jumping—that sort of thing. Continuous exercise it is not, which might account for its tradition of athletes who consume burgers, hot dogs, and beer after games.

Bodybuilding, meanwhile, is a sport that requires constant levels of difficult motion. Arnold Schwarzenegger in his heyday would spend eight hours in the gym every day, in addition to working in construction. Bodybuilders lift insane amounts of weight, often in the hundreds of pounds, over and over again.

In order for bodybuilders to gain the level of muscle required for their job, they need to eat a lot. And like, *a lot*. Thousands and thousands of calories more than you or me. In fact, it's not uncommon for bodybuilders to wake up multiple times a night in order to force-feed themselves entire chickens before going back to sleep.

What I am saying here is, the type of sport an athlete plays is going to influence their dietary choices. Intermittent fasting, then, might work for some more than others. For bodybuilders, there is a zero percent chance that this will be beneficial, because of the demands of the sport.

This actually goes for endurance athletes in general, including marathon runners. Running a marathon is, for how common a practice it's become, an insane thing to do. You are running so far. Because of this, many runners actually have difficulty getting enough fuel in their bodies to accomplish these feats. It's not unheard of for runners to eat every two to three hours, similar to bodybuilders, although with different goals.

Should runners try intermittent fasting then? Probably not. Remember, part of what we are doing here is trying to lose weight and stay healthy, possibly by changing our relationship to food. This is not really a problem among marathon runners, who tend to be in insanely good shape anyway. (Even though their knees might occasionally disagree with them.) Even if they think they could use a change in their relationship to food, it'll be at the cost of being able to run a marathon. So that is a choice you can make, but there are probably better options out there.

But let's say you are an athlete and you really, really want to give this a try. One of the things you might benefit from is a slight change in the eating window. If you are an athlete and you are interested in the 16:8 protocol, why not try 14:10? That extra two hours might do you a lot of good. In fact, it could mean a whole extra meal.

Remember, it's not uncommon for athletes to eat more than three meals a day. Maybe this means eating smaller meals more often, or maybe, if you are a powerlifter, it means eating several enormous, gut-busting meals, over and over again. An extra meal can be the difference between winning and losing, and, in athletics, that is everything.

In fact, a lot of us will be familiar with the phrase "carb-loading," which is what athletes do to make sure they have adequate energy to perform. Essentially, this is where they eat a boatload of carbs, like, say, enormous bowls of pasta, in order to have high glycogen levels. Those glycogen levels are important because that is where our energy comes from.

For us non-athletes, burning through glycogen is a good thing. It means we are burning fat. But fat is stored energy! And athletes, I do not know if you know, generally do not have much in the way of fat on them.

They need those carbs in their system. They need the fuel, because they are going to attempt some crazy maneuvers to make their living. Not only running long distances but hitting things—or people—very hard. Every calorie counts with athletics, and cutting back on the amount of fuel you put into your body is likely going to cost you.

Unless, of course, you want to shovel those calories into you over smaller periods of time. But there is no way that is good for you, so my advice would be not to do that at all.

In fact, what is known as intuitive eating might be better for athletes overall. This means that you do not eat at scheduled times, but instead eat when you are hungry and stop when you are full. Intermittent fasting by its nature is the opposite of this since you have periods where you are super hungry and do not eat a damn thing.

If you are interested in intuitive eating, there is lots of research out there on its benefits and drawbacks. But for now, we'll just have to flag it as a point of potential interest, because, alas, we have to get back to the subject of this book.

Now, where were we? Right, athletes. Okay, we are returning again to the athlete who really, really wants to give intermittent fasting a try. Are there any benefits to doing it?

The answer is: "maybe." I know, not the best answer. But there is some evidence that fasting might be good for a couple things, namely giving your body more recovery time, and getting your circadian rhythm on track.

Regarding recovery time, there is some evidence that the 14:10 window might actually help with that. Why this is might have something to do with how intermittent fasting affects sleep, in that some study participants have said that they sleep better while on that protocol (Santilli, 2020).

Sleep, as we know, is one of the key ingredients to recovery after a workout. That is when our body does most of the repairing, which means muscle is being built.

Anyone who's ever worked out and gotten a rough night's sleep after knows how much of a drag that can be too. Everything hurts! So, adopting a procedure that allows for deeper, more restful sleep is going to be something of a godsend.

All of which, of course, ties into your circadian rhythm. Problems with this are causally related to elevated levels of stress, which can have an enormous impact on your physical health. Mind and body are, after all, deeply connected. Putting yourself on an eating schedule, and a sleeping schedule, can help regulate your circadian rhythms, which in turn helps you sleep better, which in turn helps you recover better.

By the way, for those of you wondering what your circadian rhythm is, it's your body's internal 24-hour clock. We have a sense of how long our days are, which also means how long our nights are. If this goes out of whack, as you can imagine, we are in trouble.

So, what is the verdict, then?

Well, it appears as though the jury's still out for athletes, doesn't it? There are a bunch of factors at play here, most of which stem from which sport the athlete plays. But in general, how can we expect someone who needs to take in a high number of calories to limit the time over which those calories are taken in?

The truth is, we can't. Which means that when we are considering intermittent fasting, we have to pay attention to what our lifestyles are to see if it fits. This program is not, in other words, a one-size-fits-all. There are mitigating factors here.

Extrapolating from this, we might look at other career choices, in addition to lifestyle ones, to see if maybe fasting might be a detriment to us. This has been mentioned before, but what if we work a job where our minds need to be sharp? Maybe we try fasting and find that we get all loopy without food. Is fasting the right call for us, then?

Bodies, as they say, are different. Needs are different, the same as goals and everything else. Being attuned to what works best for you based on these factors is going to be to your benefit. Usually that means experimenting, but it also means doing research and talking to your doctor or dietician—lots of things.

Just remember that if intermittent fasting doesn't work for you, then you have plenty of other options. That includes the traditional route of diet and exercise, among others. So do not get discouraged. We really are all different!

And speaking of different, let's get into the fraught area of sex differences in biology, what that means for nutrition, and whether or not fasting outcomes are different for men and women.

Men and Women: Biology and Fasting

As a caveat here, I understand that this is a contentious issue at the moment. The culture war has reared its ugly head and the battle over biology has come to the fore. My intention in this section is not to cast my lot in with one side of this debate or the other, nor any of the myriad millions of permutations in between. My intention is only to talk about biology, how nutrition affects that, and how it should influence our decisions going forward regarding whether or not to adopt intermittent fasting.

With those parameters set, then, I think we can move into this section smoothly, calmly, and without assuming bad faith on anyone's part.

The first thing we'll notice when looking over the literature is that the nutritional needs of men and women are very different from one other. And this is an important thing to know! It means that food affects men and women differently, and in a variety of ways.

Let's just start with calories. For men, it's generally expected that you'll need between 2,000 and 3,200 calories per day. For women, it's between 1,600 and 2,400 per day. The reason for this is that calorie needs are dependent on the size of the person, including how much they weigh. Men tend to weigh more than women, so they need more calories.

Calorie needs are also dependent on things like age and activity levels. So, as we said earlier, athletes need to take in more calories than non-athletes. But so do construction workers and other laborers. And, obviously, adults need more than infants.

Muscle mass and overall size influence what our protein needs are. While it's extremely difficult to adopt a diet that limits our protein intake, considering how ubiquitous it is, nonetheless it's true that larger, more active people do need more protein than smaller people. And this means, yes, that generally speaking, men need more protein than women.

This will be obvious, I think, when looking at the bodies of male and female bodybuilders. Female bodybuilders can, no doubt, achieve an enormous size. But the sheer gigantism of a body like that of Greg Kovacs, who, in his prime, reached over 400 lbs., is almost beyond comprehension.

A body like that, or like Arnold Schwarzenegger or Lou Ferrigno's, will need more material in order to be maintained. And that includes protein. In fact, without protein—and a thousand other things—none of those athletes would have been able to reach that size.

Fiber is another important dietary input with different sex-based variables. To begin with, it should be said that most Americans do not get enough. That means more of us should be eating fruits, vegetables, nuts, and seeds. See, what it is, is indigestible plant material. Because we can't digest it, it helps move our digestion along. Without it, we run into digestive problems, which makes us unhealthy.

In fact, most Americans eat only 10–15 g of fiber per day. But the recommendation is 25 g for women and 38 g for men. So, most of us are way, way off (Lappe, 2023).

But notice here, as elsewhere, that the nutritional needs of women and men are different from one another. Men require more fiber than women, which means they should be eating more fruits and vegetables, even more so than their female counterparts. The body has needs, those needs vary across populations, and this is an important one to note.

That being said, none may be more important to take note of than water. You'd think, with how important water is, that we would be good at drinking it. But no. We must be a dehydrated people, because the amount of water we drink appears to be constantly under the recommended daily intake.

First of all, it's key to up how much water you drink in proportion to how much fiber you ingest. So, as we eat more fiber, we want to drink more water. For women, this means drinking roughly eight cups of water a day, or nine if they are pregnant. For men, this is about ten cups a day.

That might seem like a lot of water but remember that this is throughout the day. Me, I tend to drink carbonated water with one of those fantastic SodaStream things. I would say it helps me go through about six to eight liters of water per day. But that is just me!

Okay. I think we have noticed the pattern by now, but there is one more point that is crucial to make. And that is to do with alcohol.

Alcohol is a mixed bag even on a good day. There are some benefits from drinking in moderation, although the current research on its cancer-causing elements might overwhelm that sooner or later. It can be the source of good times and bad, of fun and terror. It's as ambiguous a drug as any you'll ever find.

It's also full of calories. This has to do with the sugar that produces the ethanol, which is only worse in cocktails. Beer too is loaded with empty calories. So drinking is responsible for weight gain in people, which is inadvisable if that is what we are trying to do the opposite of.

The difference between men and women regarding their recommended intake of alcohol is stark. For women, the recommendation is no more than one drink per day. For men, it's two. Body size has a lot to do with this, as anyone who's gone on a bender with a large man can attest to. (Or a small one, for that matter.)

Men can drink twice the amount of alcohol as women for the same level of consequences—generally speaking. Men are also more prone to alcoholism, so maybe that data will change in time also. In the meantime, though, it's worth noting that body size is a factor in being able to process alcohol with minimal harm, which means that our biology is key not just in taking in what is healthy, but also what is unhealthy.

I'll get back to fasting in a second. But the point of all this was to lay the groundwork for that, so we are aware of what phenotypes have to say about our diet. Bigger, smaller, male, female, these are all things to take into consideration when adopting a diet or lifestyle choice. Fasting is no different.

Now that we have got that behind us, let's get into how intermittent fasting affects men and women differently.

To begin with, some research has shown that the practice may not be beneficial for women in the same way it is for men. There is a study that showed women's blood sugar control worsened after fasting, for example. And there are anecdotal accounts of menstrual cycles being interfered with in undesirable ways too (Coyle, 2018).

The reason for this may be simple: Women are extremely sensitive to calorie restriction. What happens when women fast is that the reproductive hormones in the hypothalamus are affected, and the ones that need to reach the ovaries have trouble getting there. Hence, issues with the menstrual cycle.

Now, this does not mean that women should refrain from the practice altogether. What it does mean is that if they want to do it, it may be wise to adopt a different approach than some of the ones we have discussed earlier; say, fasting for fewer days or shorter periods of time.

There are other areas where the benefits for men and women are the same. Heart health might be one, judging by some of the research. This is because fasting seems to affect cholesterol and lower blood pressure, although more research is needed. In fact, there are some studies that say fasting has no effect on either of those things. So it's a jump ball, in a way. But the ones that do suggest a link between fasting and heart health do not say that women are excluded from the findings (Coyle, 2018).

Some of the other benefits we have covered too, including reduced inflammation, longevity, and improved mental health, do not appear to be sex-specific. But again, there is a lot more research that needs to be done before we can say anything conclusively.

Remember, this is a new idea in the diet sphere. What we do not know vastly outweighs what we know, but we are getting signals from the research that some benefits are cross-sex, and that is not nothing.

Let's return to the idea of modified fasts for women. If the traditional protocols we have talked about might not work— and even then, some of them will—what types of protocols should women be thinking about when adopting the practice?

The first one is called the crescendo method. This is similar to 16:8, but you fast for between 12 and 16 hours and you do so two or three days a week. Not, it should be noted, every day, and you should do it on nonconsecutive, evenly spaced days: say, Monday, Wednesday, and Friday.

Eat Stop Eat is an option too, but for women it's advised that they fast for no more than two days per week. Also, starting with 14–16-hour fasts and then building from there will help get your feet wet without jumping into the deep end.

For 5:2 and 16:8, the recommendations for modifying are vaguely similar to what has been listed above. During the fast days for 5:2, it's advisable not to go no-calorie, but to cap off at 500 calories. And for 16:8, the recommendation is to do 14 hours of fasting instead.

So, much like how women need fewer calories per day than men, the amount of time spent fasting should be shorter also.

And even then, having some calories in there is advisable in order to maintain maximum healthiness, and thereby avoid menstrual problems and other associated issues.

If you keep this in mind as a principle, any fasting protocol you come across can be modified accordingly. No doubt there will be more of them discovered by the time this book is out, and from there, there will definitely be plenty more. But given the health risks women face when adopting a fasting protocol, it's important that they scale back the number of days and hours spent fasting, and, if possible, add roughly 500 calories to their diet on fast days.

Easy peasy. Simple as pie.

Alright, now we are not quite done here. So far, we have been trying to figure out where the limits of intermittent fasting might be. We have learned that it's not a one-size-fits-all activity, and that lifestyle choices and biology can play an inhibiting role with regards to how well the practice is going to work.

The last thing we need to look at, then, is mental health.

Fasting and Mental Health

This is a big one, folks. Mental health disorders are devastating conditions to live with. Treatment for them is only now beginning to claw its way out of the dark, which means we have come a long way since the heyday of lobotomies and diagnoses of hysteria, but there is still much, much more to learn.

For that reason, we need to be cautious here. First off, treatments for mental health conditions will evolve, and so much of what we talk about here might seem really dated really quickly. But also, treatment can be precarious and if we are undergoing treatment for our mental health, upsetting that balance is absolutely the wrong thing to do.

But we are getting ahead of ourselves. First, we are going to look into the connection between nutrition and mental health. And then we are going to get down to business and see if fasting is a good or bad idea for people with mental health conditions. All, of course, with the caveat that the best person to talk to about this is your doctor or, if you have one, your therapist.

That said, let's get to it.

We know that nutrition is important for our physical health. But given how integral our physical health is to our mental health, the next logical step is to connect food and mood, although preferably in a way that doesn't rhyme as clumsily. So, what are the specific ways in which our eating habits affect our mental health?

Well, scientists have developed a kind of three-pronged approach to study this. First, there are the ways in which dietary patterns affect mental health. Second, there is the biochemical level of nutrition. And finally, there is what is known as gut and brain health.

One study published at Harvard looked at people whose diet was either what we would call "Mediterranean" or "traditional Japanese." These people's mental health was compared to those who ate what we might think of as the "Western" diet, which is made up of huge portions of, often, meat and fried rubbish, with few vegetables (Caton, 2018).

Well, guess what? Those who followed the Mediterranean and Japanese diets had a risk of depression that was 25–35% lower than those who followed the Western diet. And as far as the researchers could tell, it had a lot to do with the amount of vegetables, seafood, lean meats, and unprocessed grains, while the Western dieters were eating processed, sugary, fatty, salty nonsense (Caton, 2018).

Now, just to make a note here, we all know that correlation does not equal causation. Or, at least, I think we do. And if we do not, then we do now.

Anyway, there could be other mitigating factors that led to such a huge discrepancy. But there does seem to be some level of relationship between our food intake and our mental health. And luckily for us, this is not the only study that produced this result.

This one, in fact, is super interesting. It comes out of Australia and was set up as follows: Half of the participants were asked to follow the Mediterranean diet, and half were put in a social support group. The idea was to monitor depressive symptoms in both groups and see which environment had more of an effect (Caton, 2018).

The perhaps shocking result was that the group of dieters fared better than those in the social support group. And by a bit too. In fact, a third of the people who followed the Mediterranean diet were more likely to enter a remission from major depression (Caton, 2018).

Is that not crazy to you?

Put together, these two studies do appear to say that the connection between diet and mental health is strong. Not to the extent that diet is a cure-all for depressive symptoms, because obviously depression is a multifaceted illness. But there is the takeaway here that our mental health can, it appears, be strongly affected by our diet.

This should perhaps make us slightly cautious about fasting, then, if we have major depressive disorder. After all, if our diet and mood are that strongly connected, then what happens if we throw a wrench in the gears? Are we going to make our symptoms worse?

Luckily for us, there is some research on this issue. And while the overall results are currently ambiguous, there are reasons to be optimistic.

On the one hand, we have a review from 2021 on the effect fasting had on depression and anxiety. This review came from five randomized controlled trials, which are the gold standard in research. It found that people who fasted were less likely to experience symptoms of depression and anxiety than people who did not (Fishman, 2022).

But there is another side to this, this time from a more recent review in 2022. This one found that fasting was likely to induce negative emotions like irritability—remember, those of us prone to angriness are going to have a tough time with the practice. But at the same time, the review found that there were positive emotional outcomes, like a sense of accomplishment (Fishman, 2022). So, this one's more ambiguous overall.

Which one are we to believe, then? Well, "both and neither" is probably the responsible answer. But we can dig a little deeper into the pros and cons and, with any luck, learn enough to at least make our decisions well-informed ones.

Since one of our goals here is weight loss, many of us reading this, right now, will know the effect that weight gain can have on our mental health. For lack of a better phrase, it sucks. Our self-image goes down the toilet, our self-consciousness goes way up—it's quite the state to be in.

If fasting does help us reach our weight loss goals, then it will, by definition, help ease our mental distress. With the caveat, as always, that there is a well-established connection between fasting and certain types of eating disorders, indulging in which will only cause mental distress. So, it's a double-edged sword: If done in a way that is healthy and nonpathological, fasting can lead to outcomes that will make us feel better; done in a different way, it can be both a cause and symptom of something that has gone wrong.

Another thing we have talked a lot about is how fasting affects our metabolism. But this too has an impact on our mental health! Because it turns out that the anti-inflammatory response that is caused by metabolic changes also helps us resist stress, which in turn lowers our anxiety levels. Hence, good for our mental health (Fishman, 2022).

And the thing about anxiety too is that it seems to be on the rise in virtually every corner of Western civilization. In fact, it's hard to find someone who doesn't claim to be struggling with their anxiety on some level. Which is not just concerning in itself, but anxiety is also linked to a whole host of secondary effects, including cancer.

Reducing the overall level of anxiety in this part of the world would certainly do us a lot of good. So, is it worth thinking about intermittent fasting as a way to possibly mitigate the effects of anxiety on our population?

Well, let's not move so quickly. For all that we have covered here, the picture of fasting's impact on mental health seems to be a both/and approach. For example, fasting is also positively correlated with feelings of depression and anxiety, as well as anger and fatigue (Fishman, 2022).

So, why does this happen? Well, nobody really knows. The going theory seems to be that blood sugar levels have an effect, but the jury, so far as I know, is still out. Nonetheless, it is true for some people, and for that reason fasting is not an easy recommendation for people struggling with these states to begin with.

But, of course, there is the complicating factor. Because at the same time, a 2016 study on healthy women found that fasting gave them a sense of achievement, reward, pride, and control. And among Muslim practitioners of fasting over Ramadan, there are reports of them gaining an overall sense of psychological well-being, self-acceptance, autonomy, and personal growth (Fishman, 2022). All of which are feelings that would, by their nature, counter feelings of depression.

So, which is it? Is it good for our mental health, or is it bad? Are we just throwing dice when we mix poor mental health with fasting? Or is there some X factor that we are missing?

Knowing that our physical and mental health are connected, we might find an answer by looking at the physical symptoms associated with fasting. For example, when we are fasting, we are not taking in calories; calories are energy; no energy means we experience fatigue. Fatigue, as it happens, is also associated with depression.

Coming off a fast is also associated with overeating. Overeating in itself is going to make us unhealthy and possibly make us feel depressed either because a) we have lost control of our weight; or b) we are ashamed of our inability to control our eating habits.

And what about nutritional deficiencies? If, when we come off a fast, we eat nothing but junk, how is our body going to produce the hormones and neurotransmitters necessary to balance our mood?

Is it possible, then, that keeping ourselves healthy when undertaking a fast—meaning we eat well when we need to, take the right supplements, make realistic plans that we stick to, and adjust those plans based on our biology—will help stave off the effects of depression and anxiety that might otherwise be a direct result of the practice?

One element we might notice among the positive findings above is that fasting during Ramadan had an especially high rate of positive feelings associated with it. Ramadan is, crucially, a religious undertaking. That means there are religious and spiritual feelings and goals that are being added to the mix and are therefore missing among people who are fasting for weight loss, just as an example.

Could it be, then, that what we bring to the fast mentally has an influence on our mental health outcomes? We have already talked about how fasting can be a symptom of an eating disorder. In that way, what we expect to get out of it—in that case, an unobtainable appearance that conforms to our pathological self-image—in some sense pollutes the practice right off the bat.

Let's bring in another example here and see what we can learn from it.

Mindset and Fasting

One of the great religious writers in the history of the world is the formidable St Augustine. He was, in brief, a North African in the Roman Empire who went through a period of spiritual seeking that lasted until his 30s, when he found Christianity. He later became a bishop, but he's mostly known for his books, sermons, and commentaries, which influenced the direction of Western Christianity for roughly a thousand years (and still affects it today).

In his Sermon LXXII, this is how he describes the effects of the practice (Augustine, 2016):

> Fasting cleanses the soul, raises the mind, subjects one's flesh to the spirit, renders the heart contrite and humble, scatters the clouds of concupiscence, quenches the fire of lust, and kindles the true light of chastity. Enter again into yourself.

Okay, fancy talk there. But what does it mean?

For Augustine, the "passions," or body desires, were meant to be subjected to reason, or "spirit." The goal of the spiritual life was to conquer these desires through practice, which involved prayer, meditation, reading, and ascetic practices like, yes, fasting.

"Practice" here has been used in two senses: one, in the sense of "ritual practice," as something that is done; and two, in the sense of "practice makes perfect," or doing something repeatedly until you have mastered it. It's the second sense of "practice," however, that is going to be crucial for us.

Augustine was like you or me, in that he was only human. In fact, if you have ever read his work, you'll know that he was very, very human. He enjoyed partying and carousing, could be quite vain, and fathered a child out of wedlock with a mistress he kept. In other words, he knew the passions well.

During a fast, then, he would have experienced all the things that you or I do. He would have felt hunger, irritability, annoyance, the whole gamut. It would have been as hard for him as for anyone else.

But what the fast does, as he says in the quote, is allow him to conquer his body. His stomach whines at him, and he says, "Not yet." His body grows tired, and he says, "When I am ready." It's a period of trial, in other words, that provides an opportunity for spiritual growth and the mastery of the body by the mind. He practices facing the adversity of the body and, with enough time, manages to overcome it.

I know, I know. More fancy talk. But also notice here that his expectations going in are already nonpathological. He is not expecting something unrealistic or undertaking a fast because of some level of disordered thinking, for example. He's doing it because he knows it can be used as a tool for growth, and then, in using it that way, accomplishes his goals.

The question here, which is almost unanswerable, is: If our pathological expectations "pollute," in some sense, what we get out of the practice, does it go the other way too? If we go in with good intentions, in other words, do we make it more likely that we get good results?

As I said, it's probably an unanswerable question. It's not exactly the kind of thing that can be studied or falsified or anything else, which means it's not ripe for scientific study. But since we are concerned here with mental health outcomes, i.e., whether fasting eases or worsens symptoms of mental distress, maybe this is enough to signal to us that we should consider why we want to fast and what we hope to get out of it, in order to mitigate the negative side effects.

If we go in like St Augustine, hoping to use it as a period of trial to be overcome, then maybe that sense of accomplishment Muslim fasters reported during Ramadan could be at our doorstep. And if there is one thing depression can't stand, it's that.

Okay. We have made it to the end of a long chapter. How can we sum all of this up?

In Conclusion

Nothing about intermittent fasting is a sure thing for every person. There are some people, as we have seen, who would not benefit from it at all, or who would benefit from a modified version of it.

Athletes by and large have unique dietary needs that make fasting unreasonable for them. And female biology is no different—in fact, women seem to benefit more from scaled-back versions of fasting, due to the general difference in body mass between men and women.

But the point of all of this is that our goals are what matter. And when we are considering an approach to our health like intermittent fasting, it's important to make sure that it'll help us get to where we want, without doing damage to our bodies. That means not just taking our careers and biology into account, but also ensuring that our intentions are not the result of, say, an eating disorder.

That being said, what if we understand fasting as a means to give our bodies a break, to help sharpen our minds, scale back on the unnecessary calories, and retrain our relationship with food? Then maybe we'll get the most out of this practice after all.

Alright. With that out of the way, then, let's get into which obstacles we might encounter and what to do about them.

Chapter 7:

Troubleshooting Intermittent

Fasting

So here we are, nearing the end.

We have covered a lot of ground already. We have learned how to make plans and stick to them. We have learned too how to make sure we stay healthy through nutrition. We have even gone over what might be the mental and spiritual benefits of taking up fasting as a practice.

And through all of that we have learned, I think, that fasting is not easy. There are some genuine challenges to getting through even one fast, let alone doing it multiple times. How those enthusiasts who go five days without eating pull it off, I'll never know.

To end our journey, then, we'll need to go over some of these difficulties in detail. Because no matter what we do, we are going to encounter them. We are going to find ourselves hungry, lightheaded, the works. And when we do, we are going to need to have plans in mind for how to overcome them. Because if we do not have some idea of what to do, we are going to be overwhelmed and, alas, we are going to give up.

So, what are some of the most common difficulties encountered during a fast?

Some Common Difficulties

The first one is perhaps the most obvious: hunger. We feel it throughout the day normally when our body knows it's time to eat a meal. Our stomach growls, we feel a craving for food. We all know what it's like to desire to eat.

That gets multiplied, obviously, when you put off eating for extended periods of time. Your body recognizes that it has gone into a calorie deficiency, and it sends signals that it needs to eat. This accounts for the usual symptoms, including the growling stomach.

Now, funnily enough, there is a study that confirms this. Why this study ever needed to be done, God only knows. What the study did was pair intermittent fasters with people on regular calorie-restricted diets. Intermittent fasters, they found, scored higher for hunger than the other group. So, to the surprise of literally nobody, intermittent fasting makes you hungrier than plain old restricting your calories (Kubala, 2023a).

What is interesting, and useful for our purposes, is a separate 2020 study that took 1,422 people, all of whom were on fasts lasting 4–21 days. What the researchers found was that while hunger pains were common in the early stages of fasting, they abated once the body got used to the new regimen (Kubala, 2023a). This is worth coming back to, but for now let it be known that everyone who fasts, especially in the early periods, is going to feel hungry.

Less common, but perhaps more unruly, are the headaches and lightheadedness. Now, sure, everyone's had a headache before. We have all been sick, for example—or, I think we have. If it's just me, I would appreciate knowing.

But we have all been sick and we have all had headaches. Most of us have had hangovers or bumped our skulls on something hard. We know what this is like.

None of that, however, makes having a headache any more bearable. It sucks. And, unfortunately, getting a headache is something we may have to look forward to, especially during the first few days of our protocol.

Some interesting facts: Fasting headaches tend to be in the front region of the brain and of mild to moderate intensity. They seem to be more common in people who are already prone to headaches and may, in part, be because of caffeine withdrawal (Kubala, 2023a).

So, if you are someone who already gets headaches and plans on using the fasting period to come off coffee, there is a good to fair chance you are going to be in trouble. Probably. None of this is a guarantee, but if you have a low tolerance for this sort of thing and it does come in, the temptation is going to be to break the fast and get rid of the damn headache as quickly as possible.

In addition to the headaches, though, there is the possibility of digestive issues. Not just nausea either—anyone who's unexpectedly missed a couple of meals knows that nausea is a common side effect of not eating. But with intermittent fasting, there is the possibility you might develop either diarrhea or constipation.

That almost doesn't seem possible, right? How can the same thing produce two opposite symptoms—diarrhea and constipation?

Well, partly, as always, it depends on the body. But in addition to this, how you fast has an impact on what the symptoms are. Dehydration, for example, can make you constipated, because you do not have enough fluid in your body to—well, you get the idea. But in some people too, a change in diet might make them bloated, and with that comes diarrhea.

The obvious solutions to this are, then, to drink plenty of water and, when not fasting, to eat plenty of fibrous foods. If you do not, this could be your future.

But then it could be anyway! If you know your body well enough to know what dietary changes do, and you know this is a side effect for you, then you'd be wise to anticipate it once you adopt the practice. Every body is different. Knowing yours is going to be a big help.

For example, what happens, you should ask yourself, to your mood when you do not get enough food?

That was a clumsy way of putting it, but you get the idea. Hypoglycemia is a real phenomenon and, on top of being ruthlessly annoying to go through, is visited ten-fold upon anyone in close proximity. Blood sugar drops, the mood goes down, and with it all sense of patience and decorum.

If this happens to you normally, then this will almost certainly happen to you during intermittent fasting. Interestingly, though, one study found that women are more likely to be irritable during a fast. This, despite the fact that women were also more likely to come out of one with a sense of pride and accomplishment (Kubala, 2023a). So, returning again to differences in biology, if you are a woman then this is something to anticipate, on top of everything else.

But what the heck are you supposed to do about it? We all get irritable from time to time. And the rough thing about feeling like that is that it can be all-consuming. It can be almost impossible, in other words, to see past our own anger and maintain rationality.

We are going to go through some ways of dealing with this later. But for now, let's leave it at this: Almost nobody has an easy time controlling their anger when it boils up. It takes practice. This is why states have different punishments for people who wind up committing crimes in an uncontrollable rage, if it's apparent that anyone else in their circumstances would have had a difficult time maintaining their composure.

Not, of course, that we are going to kill someone because we are fasting. At least, I do not think so. Rather, the point I am making is that anger is a challenging emotion, and none more so than when it's brought on by low blood sugar. So, it's not something to dread necessarily, but it is something to think about.

A couple other things we have already covered, but which bear repeating: Firstly, that without calories we become fatigued. And if we work a job or live a life that requires us to be energetic and able to give our full attention to something, then we'll want to prepare for this, or possibly schedule a fast for when we are not going to be at work, for example. Also, without calories we'll probably have trouble sleeping, which of course adds to fatigue. These are things you already know.

What you may not know is that fasting might give you bad breath. Yes, you read that correctly—bad breath. Many of us will be familiar with this wretched side effect if we have ever tried the keto diet, but basically what happens is the process by which your body breaks down fat makes the inside of your mouth smell like a Zippo lighter. Dehydration too can cause bad breath, and lots of people who try fasting wind up dehydrated.

Is bad breath the worst possible side effect? No, obviously not. But does it suck? You bet.

Consider the effect this will have on your poor romantic partner. Or, if you do not have one of those, but you are a close talker and laugh a lot, maybe you'll want to use more mouthwash or drink tons of water, which you'll want to do anyway. Something to think about.

Other than that, we already know about dehydration and malnutrition as risks, but they are also worth mentioning again. Malnutrition may not be something you'll experience directly while in the midst of a fast, but dehydration might be. And feeling dehydrated is a wretched, awful thing. So be conscious of the fact that if you are not taking in enough fluids, this could be an experience that falls right at your feet.

With all that said: We know that during a fast we are probably going to feel tired, have headaches, feel nauseous and dehydrated, have hunger pangs and bad breath, and probably be prone to anger. All of this while in the midst of trying to will ourselves into not eating.

On the one hand, nobody ever said fasting was easy. And if you thought it was, I do not know where you could have possibly gotten that idea from. On the other hand, nobody ever said it would be this hard.

Who in their right mind wouldn't just say, "Screw it," drop the fasting charade, and get back to eating regularly? If only, you might be saying, there were some techniques we could use that would make all this effort endurable.

Do I ever have news for you!

Mindfulness: A Way Forward

Mindfulness is another one of those things that seems to be everywhere. People talk about mindful eating, mindful driving; psychiatry has begun teaching mindfulness; there are even, if you can believe it, mindfulness cults out there.

But what is it? How does it work? And is it useful for our purposes?

First off, mindfulness is a type of meditation technique where you, appropriately, focus your attention on this, that, or the other thing. Commonly, you'll see that practicing mindful meditation means focusing on your breathing.

What does this mean? When you are meditating, you are sitting still with your eyes closed. Your brain wants to find things to think about and so you can feel your thoughts rush in to fill the sensory vacuum. Lots of people when they first try meditating find that they are flooded by negative thoughts, which can be a dispiriting experience. But in most cases the kinds of thoughts are just memories, or, maybe most commonly, worries about the things that need to be dealt with in the real world.

Focusing on your breathing helps train your mind to not be distracted. It's like working a muscle, where the more you do it, the easier it gets. Eventually, you should be able to focus your undivided attention purposefully in a non-meditative setting. Which is helpful, considering how distraction-oriented the modern world is.

What we are going to do here is focus on a few of these exercises in particular. And then we are going to talk about how to apply them to fasting.

First is an exercise called "body scanning." This is a technique that is great for dealing with anxiety. Basically, what you do is direct your awareness toward parts of your body that are feeling pain or distress, then sit with those feelings and contemplate them as deeply as you can.

The benefits to this are legion. To begin with, the practice helps reduce stress and anxiety, but also improves your pain management skills and allows for greater self-awareness (Raypole, 2022).

How it affects sleep is that meditation calms you down generally. In fact, people who meditate regularly are, in general, considerably calmer than people who do not. The calmer you are, the easier you find it to get to sleep.

This is largely the same for stress and anxiety. But for pain, the picture is slightly different. I'll go into more detail on this in a second, but for now what we need to know is that becoming more aware of our pain, especially of the chronic variety, helps change the way we think about it.

So much for the benefits. How exactly is it done?

Firstly, you'll want to sit in a comfortable position. Do not lie down, because you'll probably just fall asleep. Then you close your eyes and slowly become aware of your breathing. Keep your thoughts focused on the sensation of breathing, either when the breath touches your nose, or when your chest expands, or whatever else. Stay focused on this. Periodically you'll go off somewhere else, usually by getting lost in a thought. Then you just start again, focusing on the breath.

This is mindfulness meditation in general. To add body scanning, you'll want to direct that attention, the one that is focused on your breath, to the different areas of your body. Maybe the part of you that is in pain. Or maybe you are anxious and notice that you feel anxiety in your shoulders or your back. Focus on that.

If you do this enough times, you'll gain a valuable insight regarding the nature of pain and stress. It's sort of difficult to explain, but basically what happens to people who are anxious, say, is they become consumed by their anxiety. The anxiety takes over the totality of their thoughts.

What body scanning teaches you is that anxiety is a thought. And you, your self, if you want, are not a thought. If you are like an ocean, a thought is a wave. But a wave is not the ocean, is it?

Through this exercise, you become, in effect, separate from your thoughts. You can put yourself at a distance from them, look at them, and choose how to react to them.

Another exercise that is used to treat anxiety is called "tracking." This is a mindfulness practice that teaches you to become more aware of your surroundings—basically, to get out of your head.

This one is very, very simple. As with body scanning, you'll want to sit someplace comfortable. Take a few deep breaths to begin. But from there you'll keep your eyes open and look at objects around the room. As your eyes fall on a particular object, you'll say out loud what the object is. And then do this repeatedly until you feel calm.

As I said, and what I think should be obvious now, is that tracking helps keep your attention focused on your environment, instead of being consumed by anxious or stressful thoughts. You become more aware of the stable things around you, and not the tumult of your mind, put things into perspective, and send a message to your mind that everything is actually okay.

There are others you can try as well. For example, you might try a deep seeing exercise, where you focus on an object until the minutiae reveal themselves. Your couch, for example. How long before you start to see all the different shades and colors, the individual fibers?

You could also do a deep listening exercise, which functions the same way but with sound. What happens if you try it with your favorite music? How aware of the nuances of Katy Perry can you become?

There are a whole bunch of different ways you can approach this. But the lesson in all of them is the same: that you are not your thoughts. Pain is a thought just as much as stress and anxiety. In this way, mindfulness is a great tool for going to the dentist. Or when you are working out after adding weight to your regimen.

How, then, does this apply to fasting?

Let's think of all the things we have covered in this chapter, regarding the negative experiences we'll probably encounter. Hunger, irritability, fatigue—the whole gamut. We have said that in every one of these instances, whichever one happens to us, we are going to be tempted to break the fast in order to minimize the negative experience.

But if we try mindfulness techniques while this is happening, we might learn that all of these thoughts we are having are, in the most minimal way possible, just thoughts. We have a thought that is hunger, or fatigue. And we can let that thought come to be and pass away, noticing it on its way out, without ever letting it consume us. Just the same as anything else.

And that is not all! There are some other mindfulness techniques we can use beyond the meditative ones that might be of service to us.

For example, and this might sound strange, we can take the opportunity to be grateful for our hunger. I know, I know. People are starving all over the world. Being grateful for our hunger is like being grateful for being kidnapped. Or for losing a limb to land mines.

But consider the difference here. We are undertaking an exercise that is meant to improve our health, both body and mind. We are not actually starving, because that would mean what is happening is pathological. In fact, we can use that moment of the experience of hunger to think about the suffering of others and become more attuned, in our small way, to what it must be like to experience this in a way that is beyond our control.

Our gratitude, then, comes from knowing that this experience is a gateway to an improvement of the self and a connection with others. The pain of hunger is temporary, but the connection we develop could be revolutionary.

You can also take the time to think about what we might call "secondary nutrition." Here, as we experience hunger, or any of the other side effects of fasting, we can think about the other desires we have and how they are satisfied by things in our lives.

For example, we have "hunger" for companionship. How is that hunger satiated? By our friends? Family?

We all experience a kind of nourishment when we are around beautiful things. Art, nature, all of these things enrich our lives in ways that we might compare to satisfying a hunger. Thinking about those things during a fast might help us gain perspective on all of our other needs and how our life is made complete by many things.

But, yes, thinking about sunsets is not going to make us not hungry anymore. I get it. The hunger will still be there, until we eat something. That is one hundred percent true.

Let's return, though, to what we talked about in the previous chapter. Remember how we said that with the right attitude, and a set of nonpathological goals, we can prevent fasting from being a negative experience and turn it into a positive one? Well, this is one way we can do that.

We can take the negative things we are feeling, from how tired we are to how irritable we feel, and we can use them to gain insight into other aspects of our lives. Or the lives of others! But either way, instead of allowing our negative thoughts to consume us, and to turn the experience into a negative one, we can see through the negative and gain access to the positive.

Does that sound kind of airy? Well, then let's put it into more concrete terms. Every experience of ours, positive or negative, presents an opportunity to gain knowledge. We can let ourselves become consumed by them, or we can push through and become more knowledgeable, stronger, and better equipped to handle adversity.

Altogether then: Fasting is going to be a challenge. There will be physical and emotional effects that we are not going to enjoy, and that is inevitable. What mindfulness can help us do is put those effects into perspective. It can allow us to see them not only as fleeting, but also as insights into the experiences of others.

Not bad, right? I strongly recommend it.

Okay, so much for mindfulness. There is just one more thing to cover here and then we can get on our way.

What Do We Do When We're Not Achieving Our Goals?

No matter what our goals are, whether weight loss or anything else, some of us, some of the time, are going to find that we are not achieving them, or not as quickly as we would like. What do we do when that happens?

I mean, look, there are a million things I could recommend here. If you are not losing weight, maybe pay attention to what you are eating on your off days. If you find you can't last a whole day right off the bat, maybe start smaller and work your way up.

But the big thing to remember is that you should be thinking long term, not short term. Just because you have run into a snag in the short term doesn't mean the whole project is a failure. It just means you might have to rejig a few things or try coming at it from a different angle. And all with the knowledge that there will come a time when you figure out how to solve your problem, and then results will follow.

But if that doesn't work for you, just remember: The end of every attempt, whether it ends the way you'd hoped or not, just means that another opportunity to fail or succeed begins tomorrow. The fact that you can manage to get up every day and come at the problem head-on, which you absolutely can do, really should mean more than your results.

But if you keep trying, eventually you'll succeed. You'll become a stronger person not just for having reached your goals, but for having tried in the first place.

Or, as the great Jillian Michaels says: "It's not about perfect. It's about effort. And when you bring that effort every single day, that is where transformation happens. That is how change occurs."

In Conclusion

What have we learned over the course of this chapter, then?

What I hope we have learned is that challenges, whether in fasting or in any other aspect of our life, are not insurmountable. I mean, breathing in space is. But ones we are likely to run into here on Earth? Not so much.

Techniques are available that can help us overcome those challenges. But all of the ones we have talked about have been mental. Mindfulness is mental. Not being overcome by the fear or reality of failure is mental.

However we come at the problems associated with fasting, it's important that we begin by having a healthy mindset. Come in with determination, courage, and the tools to conquer adversity. And if we can do that, we can come out the other end with that sense of pride and accomplishment we have been talking so much about.

Conclusion and Additional Resources

Well, would you look at that.

We have arrived at the finale. We have landed on the runway, smoothly, safe, and sound. The pilot has begun taxiing and has encouraged us all to have a pleasant stay. The passengers have begun the hand clapping routine, which continues to confuse us all—including the ones participating.

The weather is warm. Pressure has equalized. And it's time to begin the slow shuffle down the aisle and back to civilization.

But what a whirlwind!

When we started this book, we knew we had a few vague goals in mind. Losing weight was an obvious one. Obesity has become such an epidemic in this part of the world that it receives near-constant attention. It's at the root of all these fad diets, for example, and therefore a source of cultural anxiety.

So of course, it's something we are interested in. We know that our health has spiraled out of control as a people. We are looking for ways to get out of the cycle and back into having a healthy body weight.

And is it just for aesthetic reasons? No. We know that having a healthy body weight is good for our minds too. Not only do we gain self-esteem from it, but by putting healthy foods into us, our brains are nourished and can function properly.

Which is, I think, one of the things we really learned. Our minds are being taken care of when we take care of our bodies. They are not separate from one another. We are an embodied creature. Our physical health is our mental health.

Intermittent fasting is one way we can help course-correct here. We have gone over all the different ways it affects our bodies, and how that affects our minds. But one of the things I think we learned throughout this book is that the practice can help us reset our relationship with food.

It can help us tell the difference between eating because we are hungry and eating because we are bored, or because we are unhappy. It can help us learn what hunger is and how to control it.

Once we learn to control our hunger, the doors have blown wide open. Our hunger is not our master anymore. And when our hunger is not our master, we are less likely to fill ourselves with unnecessary junk. We eat what we need because we need it.

What it takes is discipline.

So, let's not kid ourselves here. There is a long road ahead of us and this is not, much to my dismay, the only book you'll ever need on intermittent fasting. The amount of information out there is enough to make you dizzy. And so much of it is worth investigating.

With that in mind, I thought I would do what I think is the kindest thing a person can do and recommend a list of books. Whether you read some or all or none of them is, obviously, up to you. But as a parting gift, I can't think of anything I would rather do.

So here we go.

First off, there is a book by Jason Fung, MD, called *The Complete Guide to Fasting*. This guy helped over a thousand patients adopt intermittent fasting, and this is his book, so you know it's coming from a place of experience. In it, he details not only the history of fasting and how it works, but also gives you recipes you can try (Kaupe, 2023).

That he's a doctor should make the book all the more interesting. It's a must-have for anyone interested in the subject and a great help for anyone taking up the practice.

Next is a book by Gin Stephens called *Delay, Don't Deny: Living an Intermittent Fasting Lifestyle*. This book really drives the point home that healthy eating involves listening to your body and learning to control your eating habits—not denying yourself your favorite foods (Kaupe, 2023).

It's not only accessible in terms of its readability, but also easily found at your favorite online retailer. Stephens really backs up what she's saying too, so you do not have to worry that what you are getting is bunk. Consider this book one of the essentials. And do not be afraid to recommend it to a friend!

Next, by Michael Mosley and Mimi Spencer, is *The Fast Diet*, the #1 *New York Times* bestseller. Mosley is an interesting character, because he started off as a doctor and then became a journalist (Kaupe, 2023). So, with this one, you get the best of both worlds!

In a more recent edition, he actually deals with his firsthand experiences of fasting. That means he has a whole load of tips for how to get through a fast, as well as recipes. He specifically focused on the 5:2 diet, so if that is the one you're interested in, this is a fountain of knowledge for you.

Also, there is an in-depth discussion with regards to how men and women experience fasting differently from one another.

Which, depending on who you are and what you find interesting, might make this one worth picking up.

Here's another one from Dr Jason Fung, as well as a couple of co-writers, called *Life in the Fasting Lane*. This is a science-oriented book, but not in the sense that it will alienate non-scientists. Additionally, it has tons of information on meal plans, exercising, the whole gamut (Kaupe, 2023).

But what is especially interesting about this book is the detail it goes into with regard to the kinds of real-life challenges people face when tackling a weight loss program. We have already covered some of that here, but if you want a more in-depth analysis, this is the place to go.

And lastly, if books are not your thing (which would be weird considering you've clearly read this one through to the end), then there are hundreds of online groups and websites— wherever you get your information, you can find what you are looking for with regards to intermittent fasting.

Which is where we part ways. The plane has finished taxiing. The doors are open, and we are being ushered off into the airport.

We have come a long way on this journey together. Even had a few laughs. But more than that, I hope we have come to understand the value of making goals, making plans, and then executing those plans. Intermittent fasting was the subject of this book, yes, but more than that I think we have covered some broader life skills.

How they apply to the goal of intermittent fasting is hopefully clear to you now. Just remember, you are embarking on a challenging enterprise. But if you are doing it to become healthier, stronger, and more resilient, and you work as hard at it as you can (without hurting yourself), then there is no reason why you can't pull this off. What it takes is strength, courage, and confidence.

Do not doubt. Just do. And the results will be yours.

Congratulations on reaching the end of 'Intermittent Fasting Book'!

By coming this far, you've already taken a huge leap towards a healthier and more vibrant lifestyle.

As a way of showing appreciation for your commitment to your wellness journey, I am thrilled to offer you a fabulous bonus – a downloadable meal planner! This planner is not just a token of my gratitude, but also a valuable tool to simplify your intermittent fasting journey going forward.

With this meal planner, planning your eating windows and ensuring nutritional balance will become as easy as pie. Whether you're a seasoned intermittent-fasting devotee or just starting out, this planner will help turn your aspirations into edible action plans!

Ready to get your bonus? It's easy! Simply scan the QR code below and follow the link to download your meal planner. There's no catch, just a desire to help you continue the path to a healthier lifestyle.

Thank you once again for choosing 'Intermittent Fasting Book'. Here's to celebrating a healthier, happier you!

As we wrap up this enlightening journey through the 'Intermittent Fasting Book', I would like to take a moment to appreciate your dedication and curiosity. Reading this far is a testament to your commitment to health and wellness, and I am genuinely honored to have been a part of your journey.

By now, I'm sure you're feeling charged, ready to embark on your own intermittent fasting adventure. Courageously stepping into this new wellness frontier might feel a bit daunting, but remember, confidence comes with action. Believe in yourself because I believe in you! I trust that the knowledge equipped from this book and the handy meal planner will be your steadfast companions on the way.

As you carry these tools into your journey, I would be deeply grateful if you could take a moment to leave a review for 'The Intermittent Fasting Book'. Your thoughts, experiences and insights will not only help me to provide better resources in the future, but also inspire countless others on their path to finding a healthier lifestyle. Every single review matters and will make a real difference.

Thank you again for joining me on this remarkable journey. I can't wait to hear about your successes, joys, and the remarkable transformation that's awaiting you!

With gratitude,

Olivia Rivers

References

Adrian, J. (2019, December 17). *I tried the 5:2 fasting for a month.* Medium, jonathanoei.medium.com/i-tried-the-5-2-fasting-for-a-month-8bba805d6ce6

Augustine. *Delphi Collected Works of Saint Augustine.* Delphi, 2016.

Autophagy. (2012). Cleveland Clinic, my.clevelandclinic.org/health/articles/24058-autophagy

Bailey, E. (2021, November 30). *How the 5:2 intermittent fasting diet can help you lose weight.* Healthline. www.healthline.com/health-news/how-the-52-intermittent-fasting-diet-can-help-you-lose-weight

Berger, M. (2019, August 22). *How intermittent fasting can help lower inflammation.* Healthline. www.healthline.com/health-news/fasting-can-help-ease-inflammation-in-the-body

Bishop, S., Close, G., Moravej, H., Roberts, J., Williams, N., & Spector, T. (2018, January 11). *What supplements do scientists use, and why?* The Conversation. theconversation.com/what-supplements-do-scientists-use-and-why-87954

Brooks, S. (2023, February 24). *Feeling the effects of stress? L-tyrosine can support focus and the brain.* Bulletproof. www.bulletproof.com/supplements/aminos-enzymes/l-tyrosine-supplement-benefits-dosage/

Bulletproof Staff. (2020, October 28). *Can you take supplements while fasting? What you need to know.* Bulletproof.

www.bulletproof.com/supplements/dietary-
supplements/supplements-while-fasting/

Cadogan, S. (2023, January 4). *Intermittent fasting alters expression of genes tied to health and longevity.* Study Finds. studyfinds.org/intermittent-fasting-genes-health/

Caton, H. (2018, August 30). *The emerging link between food and mental health.* Centre for Addiction and Mental Health. www.camh.ca/en/camh-news-and-stories/the-emerging-link-between-food-and-mental-health

Citroner, G. (2022, November 11). *Intermittent fasting linked to disordered eating, other dangerous behaviors.* Healthline. www.healthline.com/health-news/intermittent-fasting-linked-to-disordered-eating-other-dangerous-behaviors

Coyle, D. (2018, July 22). *Intermittent fasting for women: A beginner's guide.* Healthline. www.healthline.com/nutrition/intermittent-fasting-for-women

Devje, S. (2023, February 6). *Vitamin D: benefits, sources, deficiencies.* Healthline. www.healthline.com/health/food-nutrition/benefits-vitamin-d

Dion, J. (n.d.) *Mindful fasting: with Emily Shaw.* Retreat Guru. blog.retreat.guru/mindful-fasting

Eenfeldt, A. (2017, September 29). *Intermittent fasting: down 42 pounds in 14 months.* Diet Doctor. www.dietdoctor.com/intermittent-fasting-14-months

Fishman, S. (2022, October 11). *Fasting and depression: Benefits and risks.* Psych Central. psychcentral.com/depression/fasting-and-depression

Gunnars, K. (2021, May 13). *10 evidence-based health benefits of intermittent fasting.* Healthline. www.healthline.com/nutrition/10-health-benefits-of-intermittent-fasting

Gunnars, K. (2023, August 29). *Intermittent fasting 101—The ultimate beginner's guide.* Healthline. www.healthline.com/nutrition/intermittent-fasting-guide

Hill, A. (2020, August 20). *How to meal plan: 23 helpful tips.* Healthline. www.healthline.com/nutrition/meal-prep-tips

Hill, A. (2022, July 5). *Eat stop eat review: Does it work for weight loss?* Healthline. www.healthline.com/nutrition/eat-stop-eat-review

Hippocrates (2015). *Delphi Complete Works of Hippocrates.* Delphi.

Hoshaw, C. (2021, February 9). *How to calm your nervous system.* Healthline. www.healthline.com/health/mind-body/give-your-nervous-system-a-break

Hoshaw, C. (2022, June 22). *32 mindfulness activities to find calm at any age.* Healthline. www.healthline.com/health/mind-body/mindfulness-activities

Is longevity determined by genetics? (2022, July 11). MedlinePlus. medlineplus.gov/genetics/understanding/traits/longevity/

Janice. (2019, September 18). *My intermittent fasting results: 16:8 fasting weight loss results 1 month.* Salads for Lunch. www.salads4lunch.com/weight-loss/my-intermittent-fasting-results/

Kaupe, A. (2023, May 12). *8 best intermittent fasting books – A full list.* 21 Day Hero. 21dayhero.com/best-intermittent-fasting-books/

Kubala, J. (2023a, February 16). *9 potential intermittent fasting side effects.* Healthline. www.healthline.com/nutrition/intermittent-fasting-side-effects

Kubala, J. (2023b, August 16). *11 best probiotic supplements of 2023, according to dietitians.* Healthline. www.healthline.com/nutrition/best-probiotic-supplement

Lappe, S. (2023, January 9). *Men vs women: Adult daily recommended nutritional values.* BistroMD. www.bistromd.com/blogs/nutrition/men-vs-women-differences-in-nutritional-requirements

Leonard, J. (2023, March 6). *Six ways to do intermittent fasting: The best methods.* Medical News Today. www.medicalnewstoday.com/articles/322293

Lett, R. (2021, September 8). *What to eat and drink while intermittent fasting.* Span. www.span.health/blog/what-to-eat-and-drink-while-intermittent-fasting

Mawer, R. (2019, December 11). *10 health and performance benefits of creatine.* Healthline. www.healthline.com/nutrition/10-benefits-of-creatine

Pahwa, R., Goyal, A., & Jialal, I. (2023, August 7). *Chronic inflammation.* StatPearls Publishing. www.ncbi.nlm.nih.gov/books/NBK493173/

Panoff, L. (2023, March 10). *What breaks a fast? Foods, drinks, and supplements.* Healthline. www.healthline.com/nutrition/what-breaks-a-fast

Panuganti, P. (2023, April 12). *Is intermittent fasting the secret to better brain health?* Scrubbing In by Baylor Scott & White Health. www.bswhealth.com/blog/intermittent-fasting-brain-health

Pilon, B. (2017). *Eat Stop Eat: Intermittent Fasting for Health and Weight Loss.*

Quote by Jillian Michaels. (n.d.) Goodreads. www.goodreads.com/quotes/518651-it-s-not-about-perfect-it-s-about-effort-and-when-you

Ravindran, S. (2022, April 28). What the science says about the health benefits of vitamins and supplements. *Time.* time.com/6171584/are-vitamins-supplements-healthy/

Raypole, C. (2022, December 5). *How to do a body scan meditation (and why you should).* Healthline. www.healthline.com/health/body-scan-meditation

Santilli, M. (2020, February 28). *Top 10 things athletes should know about intermittent fasting.* Spartan Race, www.spartan.com/blogs/unbreakable-nutrition/intermittent-fasting-tips

Streit, L., & Amjera, R. (2023, August 1). *What is 16/8 intermittent fasting? A beginner's guide.* Healthline. www.healthline.com/nutrition/16-8-intermittent-fasting